What Every Woman Needs to Know About *Estrogen*

NATURAL AND TRADITIONAL THERAPIES FOR A LONGER, HEALTHIER LIFE

Karen Anne Hutchinson, M.D., and Judith Sachs

A LYNN SONBERG BOOK

PLUME

A NOTE TO THE READER:

Research about estrogen and estrogen therapy is ongoing and subject to interpretation. Although we have made all reasonable efforts to include the most up-to-date and accurate information in this book, there is no guarantee that what we know about this complex subject won't change with time. The reader should bear in mind that this book is not intended to take the place of medical advice from a trained medical professional. Readers are advised to consult a physician or other qualified health professional regarding treatment of all of their health problems or before making any major lifestyle or nutritional changes.

PLUME
Published by the Penguin Group
Penguin Books USA Inc., 375 Hudson Street, New York, New York 10014, U.S.A.
Penguin Books Ltd, 27 Wrights Lane, London W8 5TZ, England
Penguin Books Australia Ltd, Ringwood, Victoria, Australia
Penguin Books Canada Ltd, 10 Alcorn Avenue, Toronto, Ontario, Canada M4V 3B2
Penguin Books (N.Z.) Ltd, 182-190 Wairau Road, Auckland 10, New Zealand

Penguin Books Ltd, Registered Offices: Harmondsworth, Middlesex, England

First published by Plume, an imprint of Dutton Signet, a division of Penguin Books USA Inc. Published by arrangement with Lynn Sonberg Book Associates, 10 West 86th Street, New York, NY 10024.

First Printing, July, 1997
10 9 8 7 6 5 4 3 2 1

 REGISTERED TRADEMARK—MARCA REGISTRADA

LIBRARY OF CONGRESS CATALOGING-IN-PUBLICATION DATA:
Hutchinson, Karen Anne.
   What every woman needs to know about estrogen : natural and traditional therapies for a longer, healthier life / Karen Anne Hutchinson and Judith Sachs.
      p.   cm.
Includes bibliographical references and index.
   ISBN 0-452-27739-6
   1. Menopause—Hormone therapy.   2. Menopause—Popular works.   3. Menopause—Complications—Prevention.   4. Estrogen—Physiological effect.   I. Sachs, Judith.   II. Title.
RG186.H787   1997
618.1'75061—dc21

96-52948
CIP

Printed in the United States of America
Set in New Baskerville

WOMEN ASK . . .

- What can I do about night sweats and hot flashes?
- If I've always had cystic breasts, will they get worse or increase my risk of breast cancer after menopause?
- I seem to get migraines all the time now. Why? Is it true a sexual romp will help?
- Should I take hormone replacement therapy if I've had a hysterectomy?
- Is it normal to feel tired all the time?
- What credentials should a woman in midlife expect her doctor to have?
- What is my risk of developing endometrial cancer? Breast cancer?
- How much will estrogen reduce the chance of my getting a hip fracture?
- Is urinary incontinence common . . . and can estrogen help?
- Does hormone replacement therapy help alleviate depression?

Important questions get informed answers in—

What Every Woman Needs to Know About Estrogen

KAREN ANNE HUTCHINSON, M.D., is an endocrinologist and the director of medical education at Bridgeport Hospital in Bridgeport, Connecticut. She is also an assistant clinical professor of medicine at Yale University School of Medicine. Dr. Hutchinson lectures extensively on women's health topics, particularly those related to menopause, and her articles have appeared in numerous medical journals. She has also contributed chapters (as sole author or coauthor) to many medical and professional textbooks. This is her first book for a lay audience.

JUDITH SACHS is a health writer and speaker with more than twenty preventive health care books to her credit. She conducts workshops for women in midlife and is a facilitator in the Human Sexuality Program at Robert Wood Johnson Medical School, University of Medicine and Dentistry of New Jersey. Among her other books are *What Women Should Know About Menopause, The Healing Power of Sex*, and *Nature's Prozac*.

To women everywhere, who, armed with information, will make better health decisions for themselves and their loved ones.

—Karen Anne Hutchinson, M.D.

To my daughter, Mia, and my mother, Naomi, who have taught me about all ages and stages of womanhood.

—Judith Sachs

Acknowledgments

The authors gratefully acknowledge the time and help of Janine O'Leary Cobb, A Friend Indeed Publications, Inc.; Wulf Utian, M.D., and The North American Menopause Society; the Princeton YWCA; and Joan Klyhn, Werner Mendel, and the New Age Health Spa, Neversink, New York.

Contents

Foreword

I am always delighted when a patient comes to see me with a list of questions. It tells me that she is interested in a real partnership with her physician and that she wants to be included in the decision-making process, whether she is perfectly healthy and wants to stay that way, or she is concerned about a disease condition and wants to learn the best ways to manage it.

This is particularly true when it comes to the estrogen decision. When you reach menopause, there are a lot of confusing choices to sort out. For this reason, you need the knowledge to be able to talk sensibly and comfortably about a variety of issues. What about protecting your heart and bones as you age? What about staying vital and sexual? What about starting on a good program of nutrition and exercise that will reinforce whatever therapies you are employing?

Then you have to decide whether you want to start hormone replacement therapy right now, or whether it's appropriate for you to wait a few years and in the meantime use natural treatments that will help with hot flashes, vaginal dryness, and other symptoms of menopause that may trouble you.

Your physician is there to guide you, to examine your family history and your own lifestyle, and to recommend a variety of diagnostic tests on your bones and cardiovascular system, if you need them. But without your input, the decision about taking hormones is one-sided.

The only way for you to feel comfortable about the estrogen question is to know yourself—your body, mind, and spirit—and then to make a considered choice. You can always change your mind several years down the road, but it's essential that you figure out, with your physician's help, what you're going to do today to make yourself healthier.

In this book, *What Every Woman Needs to Know About Estrogen*, we present every woman with the words she needs that will help to start the doctor-patient conversation. Everything you need to know about estrogen—how it functions in the body when we're young; what happens to this hormone at menopause; how its decline and imbalance trigger a variety of complaints such as hot flashes and vaginal dryness; the safety issues surrounding hormone replacement therapy; how the therapy is administered; all about hysterectomy and oophorectomy; and how estrogen affects sexuality, depression, incontinence, and Alzheimer's disease—is thoroughly examined. We also cover innovative late-breaking news about natural ways to replace estrogen without medication.

There are no easy answers. But the questions you find here will hopefully trigger new thoughts and feelings that will lead to a productive ongoing dialogue with your doctor. Choices based on a good partnership between physician and patient are not only more equitable, but in the long run they also lead to greater motivation to get healthy and stay healthy. The estrogen decision can be part of a larger picture—it can empower you to take better charge of the rest of your life and to enjoy the confidence and strength of your decisions.

Karen A. Hutchinson, M.D.
Director of Medical Education
Bridgeport Hospital
Bridgeport, Connecticut
Assistant Clinical Professor of Medicine
Yale University School of Medicine

Chapter One

Estrogen—The Controversial Hormone

Only five or six years ago, nearly every woman of fifty who walked into her gynecologist's office was told that it was time for her to start taking hormones, those chemical messengers that travel through the body protecting the heart, bones, and many other tissues. If she still had an intact uterus, she would be prescribed HRT (hormone replacement therapy), a combination of estrogen and progesterone, and if she had no uterus, she would be given ERT (estrogen replacement therapy), or estrogen alone.

Today it is by no means a given that medication is for every woman going through menopause. The proliferation of studies of women on HRT and ERT have shown that there are certain risks and benefits on each side, and it's our responsibility as women and as good medical consumers to understand each perspective before we make our own choice.

The controversy over replacing hormones at menopause rages as hotly now as it did a quarter of a century ago. One camp proclaims that women must take HRT for twenty or thirty years to prevent an early death or a terrible old age. The other camp claims that medicating menopause—which is not a disease, but a life event—is irresponsible. To what extent are we to believe what we read or what we're told by our doctors? Everyone seems to have an opinion about menopause these days, and many of these opinions are contradictory.

If you are to make a wise choice, you need to ask appropriate questions and get a good working knowledge of all the facts. *What Every Woman Needs to Know About Estrogen* will be your guide when you are searching for the right way to phrase your concerns and formulate your own decision.

When Did Estrogen Become the Magic Word?

As baby boomers, we have always demanded the latest health information—we wanted to know how to handle PMS, how to have our babies in the most natural way, and how to eat and exercise in order to be more fit and feel better. Throughout our lives, we have been opening new doors to better health.

But menopause puts us in front of quite a different doorway. At forty-five or fifty, we feel the same as we always did, but we know that something we can't quite put our finger on is lurking on the other side of the threshold leading to our future. We want to make sure that it's a benign presence—one we can deal with for the next thirty or forty years. We want to know what we can do—whether it's hormones, diet, exercise, meditation, herbs, or a combination of all of these—to beat back the specter of old age.

Most of all, we want to know more about estrogen, that magical hormone that affects more than three hundred tissues in the body, from the reproductive organs to the heart to the bones to the skin to the brain. Our endocrine glands manufacture the secretions that are carried through the blood and lymph systems to the rest of the body, and, on instructions from the hypothalamus— the master gland deep in the brain—they perform their astounding biochemical activities. Estrogen, the hormone produced by our gonads or sex glands (the ovaries), has always been a force in our lives.

It's estrogen that determines our gender before we're born, and that protects our heart and bones throughout childhood, adolescence, and the reproductive years. It's estrogen that balances our HDL ("good") and LDL ("bad") cholesterol, that keeps calcium in the bone tissue, that gives elasticity to our blood vessel walls, and that directly affects our coronary arteries, helping to keep them free of atherosclerotic plaque.

But when we reach midlife, the even flow of hormonal secretion starts getting unbalanced. Our cholesterol levels are no longer as advantageous to our heart, it's harder to keep calcium in our bones, and the number of eggs in our ovaries dwindles along with our hormones. Although we had five to six million eggs in our tiny fetal ovaries, over our life span most of these are reabsorbed into the tissue of the ovaries. By menopause, we have only a few hundred left, and very few of these are viable in terms of fertilization.

Since our supply of estrogen is also now greatly de- pleted, what do we do? One of the biggest decisions we will have to make at this time of our lives is whether to replace the hormones we no longer produce in quantity, or whether to assess our risk factors, wait several years, and make significant lifestyle changes that can affect our health and alleviate any menopausal complaints we might have.

Asking Questions So That You Can Get Answers

What Every Woman Needs to Know About Estrogen will take you through the various problems and issues surrounding the dilemma of hormone replacement therapy, and it will also address many other concerns of midlife and menopause. The book is written in question-and-answer format to give you the actual words you'll need when you're sitting in your physician's office and feel confused or rushed.

You will undoubtedly want to know what to say when you have an examination and don't understand the results, when your doctor prescribes a medication or procedure and you don't really know what it's for, and when you're feeling different—not necessarily bad but unlike the way you used to feel—and can't quite explain the signs and signals your body is giving you.

You will certainly want to know what your doctor thinks about estrogen and what other authorities say on the subject. Most important, you will want to ask how *you* fit into the replacement hormone picture. Are you a good candidate or a poor one? Should you take it now or wait several years or maybe never take it?

All the questions you might think about will be addressed in the pages that follow—and they should provoke more questions, and answers, when you and your physician get together.

How Should Each Woman Make Her Own Choice?

We can't make decisions if we don't have all the facts, or if we can't interpret the facts so that they make sense to us. We read in the papers that HRT will reduce our risk of heart attack by 50 percent. But we are not told by 50 percent of what. And at the same time, we hear the terrifying news that hormone replacement may increase our risk of breast cancer and other serious illnesses. It's like being told that we can choose between getting hit by a bus or getting hit by a truck. That's not a viable choice.

The media throw a little information at us, our doctors throw a little more, and we end up with an incomplete version of the truth. No wonder we feel uncertain and mistrustful of "authorities" on menopause. No wonder only 20 percent of us who get a prescription for hormones actually fill it, and more than half of us who do start quit within one year.

The point is that data gathered from thousands of American women don't always apply personally. We must know what our *own* risks and vulnerabilities are, and then we must ask the right questions so that we can each fit our own personal puzzle together. In this book, we will supply the most up-to-date statistics, but we will also give you the tools you need to figure out whether you are right on target or above or below the national averages for risk and benefit.

Hormone replacement therapy has been shown to be very effective for most women in alleviating the signs and signals of menopause. It can wipe out hot flashes, revitalize your sex life, and give a new glow to your skin. But more important, it offers unparalleled benefits to your heart and bones—and this is really the crux of the HRT issue.

Heart disease is the number one killer of women in the United States. Osteoporosis cripples millions, not just by robbing them of bone density, but by immobilizing them so that they often have no choice but to become shut-ins. Staying in touch with the world may be the most important thing we do as humans—and these illnesses can effectively extinguish the type of social and physical contact that gives us the will to go on.

In order to keep these diseases at bay, we have to evaluate our own risk factors and decide whether we are going to choose medically prescribed hormones or natural therapies or a combination of both. We must know all we can about our personal health histories and those of our families and share this information with our physicians.

On the other hand, Dr. Isaac Schiff, past president of the North American Menopause Society and chief of obstetrics and gynecology at Massachusetts General Hospital, has said that despite the proven benefits of HRT to enhance the quality of a woman's life, it is presumptuous to suggest that every patient should take it. He asks whether it is wrongheaded to "increase the risk of breast cancer at sixty to prevent a heart attack at seventy and a hip fracture at eighty."

Every case is different, and each woman must evaluate her needs in cooperation with her physician to find answers. For example, a thin, active woman of fifty-five who has had a hysterectomy and whose father died of a heart attack at forty probably should take HRT, because she has a family history of heart disease and only requires a replacement of one hormone, estrogen. But an overweight woman of seventy who suffers from angina and has had a mastectomy to treat her breast cancer probably should not take HRT. Although she must be concerned about her heart, she has already had an estrogen-dependent cancer and therefore should probably not put more estrogen into her body. Also, since she still has a uterus, she must take estrogen plus a progestin, the hormone which creates in many users unwanted side effects and which has been shown to reduce the positive effects of estrogen on cholesterol. Thus by treating her heart condition, she could be increasing her risk of cancer recurrence.

If you are very healthy and have no family history of estrogen-dependent cancer; liver, gallbladder, or kidney disease; blood clotting disorders; or epilepsy, you are a terrific candidate for this medication. But suppose you are asthmatic, or diabetic, or you have fibroid tumors? Your doctor must help you to evaluate your condition in the light of current knowledge about HRT. And then, suppose you start the medication and get side effects? Is it worth it to live with discomfort in order to protect your heart and bones? If you have no family or personal history of risk for either condition, and you're taking care of yourself in other, nonmedical ways, can you do without HRT? After consultation with your doctor, after reading all the available materials and making sense of them, the decision is ultimately yours.

Luckily, no decision we make today is ever carved in stone. We can try natural remedies for a while to take care of existing complaints and can reevaluate our situation in a year or so. Or we can begin taking HRT and try it on for size. Maybe it will fit, maybe it won't.

In the meantime, we can learn more about our bodies, our minds, and different ways to take care of both that will stand us in good stead whether we eventually take hormones or not.

What Is Menopause?

In 1900, there were fewer than five million women in our country over the age of fifty; by 1990, the figure had risen to forty million, and now it is closer to fifty million. By the year 2016, there will be more women in this country over the age of menopause than under it. All of these women need to be reassured that they are on the right path and doing the right thing.

The first question most of them have is, What is this life event called *menopause* all about?

The word itself literally means "hiatus of the monthly cycle," and it occurs at one moment in time. It's the instant you remove your last tampon or throw away your last sanitary napkin. You may not actually know that it has occurred until you realize, after a year or so, that you haven't had a period.

The time before you experience any changes but are chronologically in midlife is called the *premenopause*. When you first experience irregular periods or start having hot flashes, you are in *perimenopause*. And finally, after you have had no menses for at least twelve consecutive months, you are *postmenopausal*.

Another concept that's important to know about is the *climacteric*, the two- to ten-year period when your hormone production becomes erratic and you may experience some physical and emotional changes. This time overlaps the years that take you from the perimenopause to the post-menopause. This Greek word that means "the rungs of the ladder" is a more apt description of the time of life you're now experiencing than *menopause*. The other rungs—adolescence, young adulthood, motherhood, the development of a career—have all led you to the top rung of this ladder, which is still to come for most of us. At this point, you have many new choices to consider. As you stand at the pinnacle, you can look back and look forward and make decisions based on your life experience and the promptings of your heart. When you achieve the stage of life that follows menopause, you may be lacking in estrogen, but you can consider yourself wise, mature, sophisticated, and worthy of respect.

What Will the Drop in Estrogen and Progesterone Mean to Me?

You may never notice the loss of your hormones. Some women simply stop menstruating, and that's their menopause. Other women, however, report dozens of symptoms, from the very common hot flashes and vaginal dryness to joint pain and sore heels, frequent urination and urinary tract infections, insomnia and early waking, allergies, unexplained bruises, migraine headaches, weight gain, chin whiskers, crawling skin, thinning hair, "funny sensations" in the head, ringing in the ears, crying jags, memory lapses, and vertigo. Any or all of these may be part of your menopause—or none of them. Your hormones are in turmoil, and your life may be as well, but it's important to remember that this stage of your life and its accompanying problems won't last forever. The signs and symptoms will lessen in frequency and intensity, and by the time you're sixty or sixty-five, with the right attitude toward aging, you will be able to create a synthesis of your old self and your new one. This will make you feel more balanced physically, emotionally, and spiritually.

What to Do to Stay Well for the Rest of Your Life

We don't necessarily need hormone replacement to be healthy. Rather, we need to eat, sleep, and function as though our lives depended on it. This means that in addition to making a decision about HRT, we also have to consume the right foods, exercise, and manage our stress.

Maybe when you were twenty, you lived on pizza, candybars, and coffee, smoked a couple of packs of cigarettes a day, drank too much on weekends, and slept only when you absolutely had to. And you got away with it! The body is incredibly resilient, and the younger you are, the easier it is to heal quickly.

But thirty years later, the story changes. Now, if you eat junk food, you may put on weight and your cholesterol and triglyceride levels skyrocket. If you don't exercise, you may get atherosclerosis and lower back pain. If you keep smoking, you'll probably find you can't breathe—or worse, that you are diagnosed with lung cancer or emphysema. If you abuse alcohol, you risk car accidents, sleep disorders, liver cancer, and in addition you can't function the next day. The body is not so forgiving at fifty.

It doesn't matter what kinds of bad habits you've acquired over the years—this is the time to start committing yourself to good ones. If you become positively addicted to your daily two-mile walk, you'll enjoy coming home to a breakfast of fresh fruit and whole grain cereal with low-fat milk. If you learn to put yourself to bed early after a half hour of yoga practice or meditation, you'll awake the next morning feeling fresh enough to meet any challenges—from bad traffic to hot flashes. Better health can evolve from many things—from a monthly chiropractic session to a sexy day in bed with your husband of thirty years to a decision to learn to play the cello. If you keep changing and moving in your life, nothing can stop you. And even if you should become ill, you will have the resources—physical, mental, and emotional—to meet the enemy head on.

Alternatives—or Complements—to Hormones

For those women who cannot take estrogen because of a strong family or personal history of cancer as well as for those women who decide that they don't want to take medication when they are perfectly well, there *are* alternatives.

In addition to maintaining a healthy lifestyle, there are dozens of natural treatments—from herbs to homeopathy to vitamin and mineral supplementation and common-sense remedies from centuries past and cultures far away.

These treatments will reduce or eliminate many menopausal symptoms. Although they have not been shown to reduce the incidence of heart or bone disease, they clearly affect the immune system—which makes you healthier and stronger to fight illness should it appear. Holistic health means treating the whole person—body, mind, and spirit—and these remedies have been reported to increase well-being even as they alleviate menopausal symptoms. Most of them—diet, exercise, supplementation, many herbs and homeopathic remedies, and mind-body therapies such as meditation, yoga, and tai chi—can also be used as complementary treatments to hormone replacement therapy. This book will detail all options—nonmedical as well as medical—for each problem we discuss.

A Dialogue with Your Doctor

If you want the best care, you have to be the best patient. This means that you should prepare yourself before you go in for a doctor's appointment. Make a list of all your concerns in order of their importance. If you're worried about chest pains, that should be your number one priority, and after that you can ask why you leak a little urine when you sneeze, or what your doctor might suggest for a dry vagina that makes sexual activity uncomfortable.

Respond to all questions truthfully, even if you aren't proud of the answers. Don't say that you run two miles a day when all you do is walk down the driveway to your mailbox; don't report that you consume two alcoholic beverages a week if you drink ten. Your doctor is your partner in health care—but she must have the facts before she can help you to help yourself.

The more you know about your family history, the more complete your chart will be. If your parents are still alive, get all the details on their health history; if not, try your aunts, uncles, and cousins to learn what predispositions you might have. This will be important when it comes time to make a choice about whether or not to take HRT.

What Are You Going to Do About Your Menopause?

Your physician is your guide and mentor in the quest for good midlife health, but ultimately, you're the only one who can make the hard choices. It's apparent that preventive care can save time, money, and serious illness in later life. But you're not clairvoyant, so how do you know what your top priorities for prevention are? Maybe your heart, maybe your bones, maybe something much more elusive, like your sense of self-esteem.

So although this book may help you decide whether or not you want to take hormones, that's not enough. You also have to decide what type of regimen you are most likely to stick to, whether to take synthetic or natural medications, whether to swallow a pill or wear a patch. You have to learn enough about hysterectomies to understand whether having your uterus—and perhaps your ovaries—removed is the right course for you. You have to put aside your embarrassment and ask questions about tough issues like incontinence and depression so that you can get the best care possible.

If you choose to make your midlife the best season you've lived so far, you must fine-tune all the facets of your health care to create a vital and active life now, one that will remain so for decades to come.

How This Book Will Help

In the chapters that follow, we will address a wide range of questions and offer answers that invite thought and a dialogue with your physician. Chapter 2 starts by explaining the process of menopause, the endocrine system, and the action of the various hormones that help to regulate your body functions. We'll make it clear how these hormones affect the heart, the bones, and the brain, and show how replacing hormones that are depleted during menopause can keep the systems healthy. In Chapter 3, we'll describe what's going on in your body and mind and detail what you can do—medically and nonmedically—to become more comfortable with the various changes that occur. Chapter 4 gets specific about the heart and bones, and makes it clear that hormone replacement can help to keep calcium in your bones and prevent osteoporosis. It can also moderate cholesterol levels and preserve blood vessel elasticity, thereby saving you from a heart attack. Since the hottest controversy rages around the advisability of taking hormones, we'll devote Chapter 5 to questions about safety and cite studies pro and con so that you can make up your own mind, in consultation with your doctor.

How do you find a good doctor to help you in this process? Chapter 6 will guide you through a rigorous examination of the person you're paying to monitor your health. In Chapter 7, we'll assist you in the process of working with your physician to find the appropriate regimen and dosage of your medication. We'll explain everything you need to know about hysterectomy and oophorectomy in Chapter 8, and will go on to detail other uses for HRT in the treatment of incontinence, Alzheimer's disease, and depression in Chapter 9. Then in Chapter 10, we'll offer a large selection of natural ways—from foods, herbs, and other sources—to get additional estrogen after menopause.

Where Do I Go from Here?

Menopause is a time of experimentation and reevaluation. It is not simply a sequence of biochemical changes, but rather a concert of physical, mental, emotional, and spiritual alterations that will cause you to think, to laugh, to worry, to cry, and sometimes to marvel at the strange plan that life has for us.

Will we really live to our hundredth birthdays? And if so, what will our lives be like? The health decisions we make now will greatly influence what happens to us thirty and forty years from now. We have a serious responsibility to make good, informed choices that will affect not only our longevity but also our quality of life.

Ask questions, get your priorities in order, and you'll have a terrific future ahead of you.

Chapter Two

What Is Estrogen and How Does It Affect My Body?

In order to understand how your body changes at menopause, you must first know some basics of body chemistry. The endocrine system—the highly integrated set of glands that send vital messages throughout the body—affects menstruation, reproduction, cardiovascular and musculoskeletal protection, and the aging process itself. Your ovaries—your source of the hormones estrogen and progesterone—are part of the endocrine system and are crucial to your good health in midlife. When you see how all the pieces fit together, you'll have a much greater appreciation of what estrogen and progesterone have done for you in the past, and how they can function for you in the future. And it may be easier to decide whether you wish to replace the hormones lost at menopause, or to take a natural course and make other changes in lifestyle, diet, exercise, and stress management that may temper your hormonal decline.

How Hormones Work

The story of your hormones began about a year before puberty, when your brain started sending messages to your ovaries. Under the stimulation of various brain hormones, the eggs, covered in sheaths called follicles inside the ovaries, started to mature. Once a month, one follicle became ripe enough to press against the ovary wall. As it ruptured, it released the egg; this is the process called ovulation. The egg then began its journey down the fallopian tube to the uterus. If it did not meet up with a sperm and become fertilized, and you didn't become pregnant, the egg and its encompassing tissue and mucus passed from your body in a period.

As you passed through your forties, the system began to slow down and the various hormonal messages became garbled. At menopause, the connection between the brain and the ovaries alters radically. You no longer have the same access to the benefits of estrogen, which you've reaped for so many years.

And those benefits were substantial. Estrogen helped to maximize the incidence of high-density lipoproteins (HDLs), the good cholesterol in the blood, and to minimize the presence of low-density lipoproteins (LDLs), the bad cholesterol. Estrogen also helped to retain blood vessel elasticity during pregnancy, making it easier to maintain regular blood pressure during that period of greatly increased blood volume. In addition, estrogen helped to keep important minerals—calcium and magnesium—within the bone tissue so that they didn't leach into the bloodstream. It supported the production of the protein, collagen, under the skin, to give us that youthful glow. It also plumped out the vaginal tissues and allowed the mucous membranes to lubricate when we were sexually aroused.

Now, as we pass through menopause, and estrogen

supplies decline, the various systems that depend on this hormone become out of balance. It's for this reason that hormone replacement therapy or a program of natural supplementation, diet, herbs, and stress management or both is worth considering.

The Female Reproductive System

The female reproductive system is a complex montage of glands, hormones, organs, and tissues. Let us see how it is set up and how it works.

You have two *ovaries* located in your pelvis, held in place by ligaments that attach them to the *uterus* and the body wall. Each ovary is sheltered by the outlying fingers, or *fimbria*, of the *fallopian tubes*. These tubes connect with the uterus, a muscular bag able to expand and contract with a pregnancy. The uterus is lined with a layer of tissue called the *endometrium*, which thickens and then is shed each month under the influence of the hormones *estrogen* and *progesterone*.

At the mouth of the uterus is a narrow passageway called the *cervix*, which leads to the vaginal barrel that is lined with deep *rugal folds*, something like the pleats of an accordion. At the opening of the *vagina* are the inner lips or *labia*, and closer to the surface, the outer labia. The *clitoris* is the small sensitive organ at the top of the *vulva*, which is the name for the entire external sexual area. Beneath it is the *urethra*, which allows for the passage of urine. The vaginal opening of a child or young girl is partly obscured by a membrane called the *hymen*, which is often broken at first intercourse. Pubic hair covers and protects the outer structures. The top of the *pubis* sits under the shelf of the pubic bone and is known as the *mound of Venus*.

The auxilliary sexual organs, of course, are the two *breasts*, each with a *nipple* surrounded by a darker area of skin called an *areola*.

The ovaries are the female sex glands, or *gonads*, and are linked to the brain and the rest of your body via secretions known as *hormones*. A hormone is a chemical messenger that delivers information from one gland to a target organ in the body. *Estrogen* and *progesterone* are the two female sex hormones, or *steroid* hormones.

All About the Menstrual Cycle

Starting at puberty, your body goes through a monthly ritual known as the menstrual cycle. You produce estrogen during the first half of your cycle, estrogen and progesterone during the second half. The secretion of these hormones causes an egg to ripen and be released from one of your ovaries, and allows the lining of your uterus—the endometrium—to thicken as preparation for housing the egg should it become fertilized. But when the egg isn't fertilized, the levels of both estrogen and progesterone fall off sharply. Without the hormonal nourishment they need to grow, both egg and endometrium slough off in the process of menstruation.

Q: How did my menstrual cycle begin?

The first trigger in your body is the hypothalamus, the master turn-on gland in the center of the brain. When you were probably about eleven or twelve, this gland sent a message to your pituitary, which controls all the other glands in the endocrine system. The pituitary then put out hormones that homed in on your ovaries, tripping the switch that got them working. Each month, under the influence of the brain hormones, the ovaries ripened an egg and produced their own hormones. When the egg failed to be fertilized, the hormone levels in the body would drop. Without hormonal stimulation, the egg and lining of the uterus would slough off, which is the experience of "having a period."

Q: How do the ovaries get the message to ripen an egg?

The chain of events is as follows: the hypothalamus produces a hormone called GnRH (gonadotropin-releasing hormone), which in turn directs your pituitary to secrete FSH (follicle-stimulating hormone) and LH (luteinizing hormone). FSH then reaches the ovaries and stimulates the follicles so that they start maturing and begin to secrete estrogen into your bloodstream. During the next two weeks, about eight or nine follicles ripen, but only one develops enough to ovulate. When this follicle reaches maturity, it pushes against the outer capsule of the ovary in preparation for ovulation. At this point, it becomes known as the Graafian follicle, named after Regnier de Graaf, a Dutch physician and anatomist of the seventeenth century who discovered this phenomenon.

Q: What happens to the egg during and after ovulation?

The pituitary cuts back on its delivery of FSH and starts producing LH. The surge in hormones causes the follicle to rupture, and as it releases its egg, the ovarian wall gives way so that the egg can burst out and pass into the fallopian tube.

Q: What happens to my hormones after ovulation?

After releasing its egg, the follicle becomes a structure known as a *corpus luteum* ("yellow body"), and it starts to secrete progesterone, the counterbalancing hormone to estrogen. Progesterone continues to build up the endometrium in anticipation of creating a home for an implanted egg.

If the egg meets with a sperm and is fertilized, the body continues its output of estrogen and progesterone in order to thicken the lining of the endometrium as a housing for the growing zygote. However, if it is not fertilized, the corpus luteum dies and stops secreting estrogen and progesterone. The lining of the uterus starts to break down since it is no longer nourished by hormonal stimulation. In a few days, the body sheds the egg, the lining, and attached tissue in the process known as menstruation.

Q: What are the two phases of the menstrual cycle?
The first is the proliferative phase, which lasts about two weeks. During this time, estrogen is the predominant hormone. The second phase is known as the luteal phase, where progesterone is dominant. This phase continues until the rapid drop-off of hormones that leads to menstruation.

Q: What is the typical length of a cycle premenopause?
The textbook number of days is twenty-eight, although there are women whose cycles normally range from every fifteen to every forty-five days.

Q: What is the typical length of a cycle in the perimenopause?
During the perimenopause, which may last up to eight years, your cycles may range from fifteen days to several months. You just never know when you're going to bleed, or whether you ever will again. After six months have passed without a period, you can be almost sure that you are menopausal, but some women continue to experience spotting or bleeding after a break of nine months or a year.

Q: What is an anovulatory cycle?
It's a cycle that takes place without ovulation occurring. This happens in puberty when you first menstruate and

then during the perimenopause, when you no longer have enough hormonal stimulation to trigger the release of an egg. When you don't ovulate, you produce no progesterone (which comes from the corpus luteum, previously the "follicle" that released the egg), and you bleed simply because estrogen has thickened the endometrium and then a withdrawal of estrogen has caused some of the lining to slough off.

In anovulatory cycles, you may bleed at any time, and it may be a good deal heavier than when you have progesterone as a mitigating hormone.

Q: What causes the irregularities in our hormones during the perimenopause?
No one is quite sure whether the hormonal changes are due to the fact that we are running out of eggs, or that our brain hormones are working harder than our ovarian hormones. But regardless of the cause, we know that FSH levels rise as estrogen levels fall, and ovulation becomes questionable. The brain pumps out more FSH as if to encourage the ovaries to put out more estrogen—but without success. In our reproductive years, FSH rarely measures over 12 MIU (micro-international units) per milliliter of blood. By the time we're in our late forties or early fifties and pass through menopause, FSH may exceed 40 MIU. (LH rises also, but not at the same rate as FSH.)

Q: When do I decide that I'm not cycling anymore?
When a year has passed without a period, you may consider that you have passed through menopause. Until this time, you should continue to use contraception if you don't want to get pregnant.

All About Estrogen and Progesterone

The two female gonadal hormones, estrogen and progesterone, are partners in a complex system of messages sent throughout your body during your reproductive years.

Q: What does estrogen do during the menstrual cycle?

It is responsible for thickening the endometrium—the lining of the uterus—to house a possible pregnancy. It elongates the glands that produce uterine secretions, also necessary to a growing fetus. In the blood, estrogen acts as a feedback mechanism, telling the brain to cut down on FSH and to stimulate the release of LH.

(In addition to its place in the menstrual cycle, estrogen affects more than three hundred tissues in the body. See below for a description of its many functions.)

Q: What does progesterone do during the menstrual cycle?

It continues to thicken the endometrium and helps the glands and blood vessels in the uterus to increase in size. This hormone helps to keep monthly bleeding on schedule and under control. (It is for this reason that some physicians prescribe progesterone supplementation—or a synthetic version of it, called progestin—for perimenopausal women who have irregular and heavy anovulatory bleeding. See Chapter 7 for a full description.)

Q: How many types of estrogen are there?

Three. Estradiol (the strongest type and the most abundant during the reproductive years), estrone (the most abundant after menopause), and estriol (the metabolic product of the two former types and the weakest form of estrogen of the three).

Q: Are there any other sources for estrogen during menopause?

Yes, the adrenal glands right over the kidney produce a hormone called androstenedione (a very weak cousin of testosterone, a male hormone), which is converted into estrone by fat and muscle tissue.

Q: What should I know about estrone?

Estrone—the major circulating estrogen during menopause—is a weaker estrogen than estradiol, which we have more of during our reproductive years. Both age and obesity increase the conversion of androstenedione to estrone. Obese women have significantly higher rates of estrone than normal-weight women, and they also have higher rates of endometrial cancer. Although we may gain more protection for our bones and heart if we have more estrone, even a weak estrogen can cause endometrial growth, so having an abundance of estrone after menopause is a mixed blessing.

Q: Are the estrogen and progesterone in my body the same as what's prescribed in hormone replacement therapy?

No. Some supplemental hormones are made from animal and plant estrogens and some are synthetic, manufactured in a laboratory. The most common estrogen supplement is taken from the estrone in horse urine; the most common progesterone is a synthetic, called a progestin. Some physicians are now prescribing natural hormones extracted from soy and Mexican wild yam plants. (See Chapter 7 for a full description of the various hormones.)

The Slowing of the Cycle: What Happens to the Hormones at Menopause

Estrogen levels plummet rapidly after menopause, and with the cessation of ovulation you produce no more progesterone. Let's examine this process as you go through menopause.

Q: Why does menstruation cease?
During the climacteric, as your supply of gonadal hormones drops dramatically, your ovaries are no longer stimulated each month to ripen an egg. Eventually, as your egg supply dwindles and you no longer experience the mid-cycle surge of hormones that would cause you to ovulate or build up the endometrium, you stop menstruating.

Q: About how old will I be when I hit menopause?
The average age is 51.4 years; however, your menopause may be at 42 or at 58. The time of your life when this event occurs varies widely depending on many factors. Menopause patterns do run in families—so if your mother or sister was particularly early or late, you may be, too. Smoking may push your menopause ahead as much as two years—another reason to cut out cigarettes. Some studies indicate that the more children you have, the later your menopause will be, but these data are mainly anecdotal. It's also been noted that women with short menstrual cycles tend to reach menopause more quickly than those with long cycles, but this information, too, has yet to be scientifically validated.

Q: How much estrogen do we lose at menopause?
Over the two to ten years of the climacteric, estrogen levels drop to about 20 percent of their peak in the reproductive years. For women who go through a surgical meno-

pause, where the ovaries are removed, estrogen loss occurs overnight, predisposing them to more severe and intense symptoms. (See Chapter 8 for a discussion of surgical menopause.)

Q: Why would my doctor want me to take supplemental hormones (HRT)?

Replacing the estrogen lost at menopause in a regimen known as hormone replacement therapy (HRT) means an extra lease on good bones, good lipid levels, and good elasticity for your blood vessels. It gives a sense of well-being by interacting with brain hormones, and it also protects the reproductive organs from atrophying. It can alleviate the temporary distress of menopausal complaints such as hot flashes, vaginal dryness, insomnia, urinary tract disorders, aching joints, sensory disturbances, and memory loss.

Q: My doctor said I had to take both estrogen and progesterone. What does the progesterone do?

The reason to supplement progesterone is to keep the lining of the uterus healthy. If you don't take a progestin or natural progesterone, you run the risk of allowing the endometrium to proliferate unchecked. A thickened lining can predispose you to growth of cancerous cells. Taking only estrogen greatly increases your risk of developing endometrial cancer, but the addition of a progestin protects against overgrowth of the uterine lining.

Q: I've had a hysterectomy. Since I have no uterus, I have no lining. Which hormones will I need to supplement?

If you have no uterus, you only need to take estrogen replacement therapy (ERT). In this situation, the use of "unopposed" estrogen is safe because you have no uterine lining to protect.

The Value of the Gonadal Hormones to Your Heart, Bones, and Brain

Estrogen and progesterone do not affect only your reproductive system. The entire body—particularly the heart, bones, and brain—benefits from hormonal output.

Q: What does estrogen do for the heart?

At least a third of estrogen's protective effect in the body centers on the balance between HDL (high-density lipoprotein) and LDL (low-density lipoprotein) cholesterol. Estrogen is a primary influence on the way the body handles lipids—the fats we produce and ingest. Estrogen keeps LDLs low and HDLs high. For this reason, we are one up on heart disease as long as we produce adequate amounts of estrogen.

Estrogen also affects the coronary arteries, which have their own estrogen receptors. These vessels supply blood to the heart itself; when they are clogged or blocked, we may be in danger of a heart attack. The hormone prevents or slows down plaque formation by blocking the incorporation of LDLs into the artery walls.

Finally, estrogen helps to keep blood vessel walls elastic and flexible, thus keeping blood pressure low. The reason we can tolerate a much higher blood volume and blood pressure when we are pregnant is that the vessels expand and contract under the influence of this hormone.

Q: What happens to my HDLs and LDLs after menopause?

As we age and produce less estrogen, the balance of good fats to bad shifts. LDL levels rise significantly; HDLs fall slightly. This dramatically increases our chance of developing heart disease.

Q: What does estrogen do for the bones?

Estrogen helps to keep a balance between the breakdown of old bone and the buildup of new bone. It keeps calcium from leaching into the bloodstream, robbing the bones of this vital mineral. During our reproductive years, this hormone prevents loss of bone mass and density and keeps the bone tissue strong enough to withstand falls, or to heal properly when fractured.

The drop of estrogen at menopause immediately compromises the bone. Without this valuable hormone, most women lose 1 to 2 percent of their bone mass within five to seven years of menopause; but some lose as much as 5 to 6 percent of their bone mass.

Q: What does estrogen do for the brain?

Estrogen interacts with beta endorphins in the brain, those neuropeptides that reduce pain and give us a sense of well-being. It is thought that a good mood and balanced emotions during the first part of the menstrual cycle can be attributed in great part to high estrogen levels. It's not until we hit the surge of progesterone midcycle that we get the classic PMS symptoms—irritability, mood swings, crying jags, etc.

Estrogen also supports plasticity of synapses and dendrites in the brain and influences areas thought to be responsible for memory. The propensity to become forgetful and "lose words" after menopause may be attributable to the decline in estrogen levels.

Estrogen affects sleep because it interacts with various neurotransmitters and hormones such as serotonin and melatonin. Serotonin is the "feel-good" compound that gives Prozac and other mood-altering drugs their effectiveness; melatonin is responsible for our awareness of light and dark and our ability to adjust our daily sleep-wake rhythms accordingly.

Q: What other functions does estrogen have in the body?

Estrogen protects the reproductive organs and keeps the vagina and uterus from atrophying. Estrogen sent to the receptors on the bladder keeps it elastic and allows it to maintain sufficient muscle tone to prevent incontinence. The hormone also keeps the urinary tract and vaginal barrel healthy, lowering the risk of both urinary and vaginal infections. It encourages lubrication during sexual arousal, thereby making sexual activity comfortable. Estrogen receptors elsewhere in the body provide lubrication to the joints and to the mucous membranes in the eyes and mouth. And it assists in keeping the collagen under the skin in order to provide that smooth, youthful look.

Q: Is it essential that I replace the estrogen I lose at menopause?

That's hard to say. You may be at higher risk for heart disease and osteoporosis—but then again, you may not be. If you do not have a strong family history of either disease, and you have few or no personal risk factors, hormone replacement therapy may not be a necessity for you right now. This is a matter to discuss with your physician. What's essential is that you maintain or establish an excellent diet, exercise, and stress management program that will last you the rest of your life and will be protective to your heart, bones, and brain.

Chapter Three

Hot Flashes and Other Changes: Can Estrogen and Alternative Therapies Help?

It is possible to find women who state categorically that they went through menopause and felt exactly the same—physically, mentally, and emotionally—as they did before "the pause." However, the great majority of women in Western societies notice some differences. Their complaints may last a few months or a few years; some experience them with great and some with lesser intensity.

The most noticeable sign or signal that the body's supply of estrogen is diminishing is the hot flash, described by one woman as "a blast of the Sahara from my scalp to my chest." Hot flashes (which to the uninitiated may feel like the first symptoms of flu) can be passing annoyances or they may severely debilitate a woman, rendering her unable to sleep because she wakes drenched with perspiration several times each night. The second classic signal, vaginal dryness, has interfered with many a sex life unnecessarily. It is particularly distressing when accompanied by itching or urinary tract infections. Irregular bleeding, disruption in sleep patterns, and weight gain are additional problems that may occur during the peri- or postmenopause.

Other symptoms, from joint pain to dry mouth to thinning hair to headaches to tingling in the extremities, are *not* figments of your imagination but real markers that show you are going through the natural process of menopausal change.

The Signs and Signals of Midlife

You may have many menopausal complaints, or none at all—and both situations are completely normal. All the signs and signals of this stage of life can be dealt with— medically or nonmedically. When you know what might occur, you can be better prepared to deal with it.

Q: What are the most common physical signals of midlife change?

Irregular menses, hot flashes, vaginal dryness, and sleep disturbances are reported by over half of all American women going through menopause.

Q: Does every woman in the world experience these signals?

Not at all. Menopause is a concept far more prevalent in Western Europe and North America than in the rest of the world. In Japan, there is no term for "hot flash," because most Japanese women never experience a deregulation in their temperature mechanism. The reason may be partly genetic, but it probably also has a lot to do with diet. The heavy emphasis on estrogenic soy products such as tempeh, tofu, and miso in this culture serves as a natural form of hormone replacement.

Similarly, in many parts of Mexico, India, and Africa, there is no expectation that an older woman might experience a distressing stage of life. In certain African tribes, women may be elevated to positions of prestige in the community once they have passed their childbearing years.

Family influences can also be very strong—and usually if your mother and sister had easy menstruation, childbirth, and menopause, you will, too.

Q: Are any of these signs or signals life-threatening?
Absolutely not. They may be annoying and debilitating, but they are not dangerous. Many can be handled with diet or exercise, some respond very well to herbs and vitamins, and many women report improvement with a regimen of hormone replacement therapy. Most of these problems pass as the dramatic hormonal swings of menopause stabilize themselves.

Q: If I have no signs or symptoms, do I need to do anything in terms of medication or alternative therapies?
A revamping of your diet, exercise, and stress management routine is a great idea no matter how you currently feel. A low-fat, high-carbohydrate, high-fiber diet can make big differences in your HDL and LDL cholesterol levels, and exercise also creates good lipid changes, in addition to giving you the edge on bone loss, high blood pressure and other forms of heart disease, and mood swings.

If you are truly concerned about your heart and bones as you age, you may consider hormone replacement as a prophylactic measure. The best candidate for HRT is a very healthy woman who is determined to live to a qualitatively excellent old age.

Q: If I'm still menstruating, is it normal to feel some of these changes already?

Yes. The perimenopause is a time when your brain and ovarian hormones are out of sync. (See Chapter 2 for a full discussion of the endocrine system and hormones.) FSH increases at a faster rate than LH, and your level of natural estrogen (estradiol) falls. The imbalance in the body's chemistry often brings on various symptoms.

Q: What lifestyle changes will make the signs and signals of menopause easier to tolerate?

The best advice is to make small changes that offer big rewards. If you know that something is bad for you—like smoking, caffeine, and too much alcohol—then use moderation or cut it out entirely. If you know something is good for you, like exercise or eight hours' sleep a night, then revamp your schedule to accommodate these excellent pursuits.

Organized stress reduction classes are available everywhere, offered through hospital community service programs, Y's, and private psychotherapists. Different methods—behavioral, cognitive, or meditative—lead to the same good effect, which is that you learn to manage the stress you have and also avoid situations that are typically stressful for you.

Another good idea is to take up an activity that has been proven over centuries to improve both body and mind. Both yoga and tai chi chuan are stress reducers and provide cardiovascular, musculoskeletal, respiratory, and immune system benefits. Courses in these two disciplines are offered in adult school classes, at Y's, and at private gyms. There are also many good tapes and books available.

Yoga, an ancient Indian meditative exercise, uses different postures to access the body's energy. The *asanas*, as the postures are called, are performed in prone, seated, and standing positions, and nearly everything in between. Using your breath to direct energy throughout the body, you learn to stretch and contract your body in specific ways for greater strength and flexibility. Yoga builds stamina and endurance; it also maintains the body's elasticity.

Tai chi chuan *(taijiquan)* is an ancient Chinese method of moving meditative exercise that is used for health, martial arts, and meditative purposes. The various "forms," or choreographed patterns from various family styles such as Yang, Chen, and Wu, must be memorized so that mind and body can act as one. It allows *chi*, or life force energy, to move through you slowly, at your own pace. (The feeling of *chi*, which exists in every living thing, is a relaxed and aware energy, quite different from the racing heart and tense muscles of Western exercise.) Tai chi also builds strength, endurance, and flexibility.

The Most Common Signs and Signals of Menopause

We will now discuss the various concerns you may have at this time of life:

- irregular bleeding
- hot flashes and night sweats
- vaginal dryness and urinary tract problems
- insomnia
- breast changes
- wrinkles
- weight gain
- other signs and signals

All About Menstrual Bleeding

Your period was the best sign you had that your reproductive system was healthy. You may have called it "the curse" or, more kindly, "your friend," but it assured you that your system was working well. Year in, year out, you bled monthly, except when you were pregnant, during lactation, and during times when you were extremely stressed. But now the bleeding is uncertain, and it's hard to figure out whether it's normal. Here are the reasons for your changes and ways to monitor the type of bleeding you're currently having.

Q: Why are my periods irregular?
During your reproductive years, your ovaries, stimulated by the hypothalamus and pituitary in the brain, ripened one egg every twenty-eight days or so. (See Chapter 2 for a full explanation of ovulation and menstruation.) However, now that you have very few viable eggs in your ovaries, and your concentrations of estrogen are low, you may not have enough hormonal stimulation on a monthly basis to ovulate, or to get the uterine lining to slough off. You may have anovulatory cycles (bleeding without ovulation when you simply lose tissue from the endometrium as hormonal levels fall), and you may have months where there is so little hormonal output, you don't slough off any tissue at all.

Q: Is it normal to bleed heavily for more than a week?
Bleeding is considered abnormal if it comes more frequently than every twenty-one days and lasts for more than ten days. Abnormal bleeding often occurs during anovulatory cycles, when your hormones are not in balance. But if you are bleeding heavily, you may have problems with fibroids, uterine lesions, polyps, or a tumor,

which must be diagnosed and treated. (For questions about bleeding while on a regimen of HRT, see Chapter 7.)

Q: What can be done to stop the flow?

If you are bleeding excessively, your doctor may wish to do an in-office invasive procedure called endometrial aspiration (see page 163) to remove some of the superficial tissue. She might then give you 10 milligrams of Provera (a synthetic progestin) for seven days to stop the bleeding. Nonsteroidal anti-inflammatory drugs (NSAIDs), like ibuprofen or naproxen, are also sometimes helpful in addition to hormones.

Once the bleeding is under control, she might give you an oral contraceptive containing estrogen with a progestin for seven to ten days to create an artificial "period," so that you can begin to bleed regularly and she can monitor the condition of your endometrium.

You might also try antihistamines (preferably the non-drowsy type), but remember that they do dry out your mucous membranes as well as control bleeding—which might aggravate vaginal dryness.

Q: What are some natural ways to regulate excessive bleeding?

Try the following remedies:

Vitamin therapy: Take vitamin A (10,000 IU twice daily).

Herbal therapy: Horsetail tea, 3 cups daily. Dong quai tea, 3 cups daily, *only* under the recommendation and supervision of a physician.

Q: What if I don't respond to drug or natural therapies?

Your doctor would do a vaginal ultrasound to examine the endometrium, using a tamponlike device that is inserted gently into the vagina. Or she might do a hysteroscopic exam, where an instrument like a very narrow telescope, linked to a monitor, is inserted into the vagina and through the cervix for examination of the uterus.

Q: Why would my doctor perform a D&C (dilatation and curettage)?

If your bleeding has not responded to drug therapy, and you are becoming severely anemic from lack of sufficient hemoglobin, your physician may perform this procedure. In a D&C, the entire uterine lining is scraped off. In some cases, the procedure cures the problem; if not, it can at least take off a lot of the overgrown endometrial tissue that may be obscuring some other underlying problem which is causing the bleeding.

Q: Does abnormal uterine bleeding mean I'll have to have a hysterectomy?

Not necessarily. A hysterectomy should be the last resort, after all other treatments have been tried.

Your New Body Chemistry: Hot Flashes and Night Sweats

When your temperature is unpredictable, it can be unsettling and uncomfortable, but you can handle the heat waves and chills if you dress appropriately, learn to breathe, and moderate the way you eat and drink. HRT can be helpful, but there are also many vitamins and minerals, herbs, and homeopathic remedies that you can use if you don't choose to take hormones.

Q: What is a hot flash and how often might I have them?

Flashing, or *vasomotor instability*, as physicians term it, is the body's response to a deregulated temperature control in the brain and dramatically shifting hormones. The reason for the flash is still not exactly clear; however, it has more to do with the changeable nature of estrogen concentration (the ratio of estradiol to estrone to estriol) than the actual level of combined estrogens left in the body.

Your number of flashes is as unique as your fingerprints. Some women have a flash every week or so; others may have them every hour on the hour. Most women have a time of day when the flashes are most prevalent (some only have them during sleep—"night sweats") and others only have them when they're awake.

Q: How likely am I to have hot flashes?
Nearly half to three-quarters of all peri- and postmenopausal American women experience them, although they are far less common in some other countries.

Q: What does a flash feel like?
Some women report that they knew they were about to have the experience before it happened. This aura, or premonition, may feel like nausea, or a tingling or pressing sensation in the head. Some women become weak in the knees and have to sit down. Others experience heart palpitations as the flash occurs.

The upper body, from the chest to the scalp, may begin to sweat profusely. You may also "flush," that is, become red as you flash. Heart rate and skin blood flow increase, although internal body temperature may drop by as much as three or four degrees as the body struggles to correct the imbalance. After the flash, the body quickly becomes chilled as it struggles to regain its normal temperature. Most flashes last about three to six minutes, although it's possible to have one that goes on for an hour.

Q: Whenever I get a hot flash, my heart pounds terribly and I feel like I can't breathe. How do I know I'm not having a heart attack?

The palpitations and air hunger are very common and probably have nothing to do with heart disease. You should, of course, consult your doctor if you have these symptoms when you *aren't* flashing. However, a heart attack is usually (but not always) signaled by a sharp searing, crushing, or strangling pain in the middle of your chest.

Q: What is a night sweat and how often might I have them?

A flash that occurs when you're sleeping is a night sweat. They can be rare occurrences for some women, but others may be awakened as many as eight or ten times a night, which leaves them groggy and disoriented the next day.

Q: What can I do about flashes and night sweats?

There are many alternatives, some medicinal, some natural:

HRT: Most women's flashes vanish or reduce in severity and number with low-dose HRT.

Clonidine (Catapres): This antihypertensive drug masks the effects of a hot flash, and many women who choose not to take HRT get relief from this drug. However, like all medications, it has its own side effects, such as constipation, drowsiness, dry mouth, and, in some instances, low blood pressure.

Exercise: Women who practice some form of aerobic exercise daily tend to flash less than those who don't. Yoga and tai chi have marked effects on the endocrine system and also control flashing in some women.

Breathing: Since temperature regulation (located in your hypothalamus in the brain) is linked to the respiratory system, the best thing we can do is get more oxygen to the brain. When we are hot and bothered, we get anxious and tend to take shallow breaths from the upper chest, raising our shoulders and sometimes gasping for air through the nose and mouth. However, studies linked paced diaphragmatic breathing to better management of hot flashes. When you start to flash, relax and inhale deeply, expanding your belly. Let the breath out slowly, contracting your belly. You will not only calm yourself but are likely to reduce your daily number of flashes.

Nutrition: Watch what you eat and drink! Alcohol, caffeine, spicy foods, and extremely hot foods can trigger flashes. Sometimes, sipping an iced drink can stop a flash in its tracks. Eat plenty of soy products (see Chapter 10) to control and limit flashing.

Try supplements: Vitamin E (up to 400 IU twice daily) has been shown to be very effective, as has vitamin B_6 (100 mg). Evening primrose oil (500 mg three times daily) or borage oil is also an often recommended remedy.

Try estrogenic herbs and plants: Ginseng, black cohosh, false unicorn, and blessed thistle are all rich in phytosterols (estrogen-like compounds) and will help with flashing. Licorice has the same properties but should *never* be used if you have hypertension. Vitex/Chaste tree (30 to 90 drops daily for a year) is recommended for women who undergo a surgical menopause. Motherwort tincture is excellent for night sweats.

Use a fan: Since so many women are going through menopause, it's become an acceptable activity. You can keep one at home and one in your purse or briefcase.

Dress in layers and wear natural fabrics: When you get hot, you can remove a jacket, shawl, or sweater; when you're chilled, you can put them back on. Put away your turtlenecks and heat-trapping polyester clothing and wear cotton, wool, and silk.

Double-sheet your bed: Depending on the number of

night sweats you have, put layers of towels beneath you and keep dry nightshirts on your bedside table. This way, when a flash hits, you can strip off the wet bedclothes, drop them on the floor, and get into something dry before you really wake up.

Keep track of your flashes: Note the times of your flashes in a pocket diary you keep with you, and see how they coincide with periods (if you still have them), foods you eat, liquids you drink, or times of extreme stress. If you can see a pattern, you can change some of the circumstances to cut down on the number of flashes.

Vaginal Dryness and Urinary Tract Problems

The vaginal area is a sensitive one, and at this time of life, it can become even more susceptible to dryness, itching, rashes, and chafing. HRT has been shown to have a beneficial effect on the vulva and vagina; and you should also consider water-based lubricants, herbs, nutritional supplementation, and exercise.

Q: Why would I experience vaginal dryness and itching?

With the decline of estrogen in your body, the environment of the vagina changes. The mucosa do not lubricate as readily, even when you're sexually aroused. You also lose epithelial cells inside the vagina. A woman of thirty may have as many as fifty or sixty layers inside; a woman of eighty may have only five layers. The thinner your skin, the more easily it becomes chafed and raw, from the ureter to the anus. You also become more susceptible to urinary and vaginal infections at this time.

Itching and burning may result from an elevation in the pH of your secretions that may bring on bacterial changes inside your vagina. The rise in alkalinity can cause a chronic discharge.

Q: What can I do about vaginal dryness and itching?

There are many solutions for these problems, some medicinal and some natural.

HRT: Hormone replacement therapy in any form will restore a great deal of vaginal tone, elasticity, and fullness. If vaginal dryness and vulval itching are your only menopausal complaints and you do not choose to take the pill or wear a patch, your doctor may prescribe an estrogen cream (Premarin or Estrace), a testosterone cream, or a natural progesterone cream to be used twice a week.

Water-based lubricants: There are several wonderful products on the market, much preferable to the old K-Y Jelly. The best ones are Astroglide, Replens, Gyne-Moistrin, and Today Personal Lubricant. They are available in most drugstores.

Natural ingredients: Use a teaspoon of nonpasteurized plain yogurt or raw egg white, inserted in the vagina, to protect against vaginal infections and to lubricate the vaginal barrel.

Take vitamins: Squeeze the contents of a vitamin E capsule directly on the vulva and massage into the vagina.

Wear nothing unnatural next to your skin: Only cotton should touch your vulva. Cut the gusset out of your pantyhose to give that area some breathing space.

Soothing baths: For an itching vulva, soak in a warm tub to which you have added some baking soda. Use plantain ointment, available in health food stores. Never use deodorant soaps, scented sprays, douches, or bath oils.

Kegel exercises: Pretend that you are on the toilet about to urinate. Imagine that you are stopping the stream; then let go. This contraction and release will teach you how to exercise the pubococcygeal muscles between the vagina and anus, as well as the sphincter muscle in the anus. By keeping the skin of this area more elastic and toned, Kegels can actually help, in combination with other treatments, to alleviate dryness and itching. This is one of the best all-around remedies for the entire vaginal/anal area.

Q: Why do I have to urinate all the time? Is there something I can do to change this pattern?

The bladder, which lies right alongside the uterus, owes much of its muscular elasticity to estrogen. At menopause, the number of estrogen receptors declines, and it's more difficult for this organ to expand and hold urine. Sometimes multiple childbirths also cause the uterus to drop and press more heavily against the bladder.

There are a variety of solutions (discussed at length in Chapter 9). HRT seems to have a beneficial effect on urinary control, but two excellent methods of treatment are *Kegel exercises* (see above) and *behavioral training (toilet drills)* where you consume a certain amount of liquid and must wait a certain number of minutes before voiding.

All About Sleeping—and Not Sleeping

It "knits up the ravell'd sleave of care" and gives us a fresh start on the next day. But at menopause, sleep is often an elusive friend. There are various ways to get to sleep without medication—and you can also find ways to relax that may replace some of your need for a full eight hours.

Q: Why can't I sleep the way I used to?

It's unclear how estrogen reacts with brain neurotransmitters such as serotonin and hormones such as melatonin to allow us to sleep. Certainly, sleep is disrupted by night sweats and waking to urinate, and after you're up, it's sometimes hard to get back to sleep. Psychological factors also come into play—if you're upset over a divorce, a loss of job, or the death of a spouse or parent, you may find it hard to drop off.

Q: What should I do when I wake in the middle of the night?

Get up and do something. Avoid activities that require lots of concentration (a serious book) or that might upset you (doing the taxes), but select an entertaining magazine or listen to music you find soothing.

You can also practice some relaxed belly breathing, taking full inhalations and exhalations, while lying on the floor or sitting in a comfortable chair.

Q: Should I take sleeping pills?

Under no circumstances should you start the vicious cycle of over-the-counter or prescription sleeping medications. Most will leave you groggy the next day, and may require increased doses over time.

There are great natural remedies for sleep:

Practice good sleep hygiene: Don't nap during the day, and get to bed and wake up at the same time each morning. This will reinforce your natural circadian rhythms that set the clock in your brain.

Drink a tryptophan cocktail: Warmed milk, with a banana mashed into it if you like, will release the amino acid tryptophan, which is a natural muscle relaxant and sleep inducer.

Herbal insomnia cures: Try an infusion of yellow melilot (1 teaspoon herb to 1 cup of water). You might also try a dropperful of Saint-John's-wort or valerian drops in a half-glass of water, a cup of hops tea, or hops sewn into a hand-size pillow, which you can place inside the pillowcase of your usual bed pillow. (You don't have to lie directly on top of it to get the benefit.)

All About Breasts

Although your other sexual organs are hidden, your breasts are always visible and can be a source of either pride or embarrassment (sometimes both) throughout your life span. They do change at menopause, for a variety of reasons, and they should always be monitored closely, with monthly exams.

Q: Why don't my breasts stand up as they used to?
Older breasts tend to sit lower on the chest because the muscles and ligaments that keep fat under the skin lose their tone and resilience as you age. The milk glands also shrink, and the breast becomes more fatty and less fibrous.

Q: I've always had cystic breasts. Does this mean I'll get breast cancer after menopause?
Certainly not. Remember that the new adjustments in your hormones may make a benign lump more pronounced at certain times. If you are uncertain about what you're feeling when you do your monthly breast self-exam, contact your physician immediately.

Q: How should I do a monthly breast exam?
If you are still having regular periods, you can examine your breasts on the second day after your flow stops. If you have no periods, or if they're irregular, do the exam on the first day of each month.

Examine yourself once in the shower, when your skin is slippery and easy to move, and then once dry, standing in front of a mirror so that you can also see the breasts. Begin by feeling around the whole breast area, from the glands under the armpit, up beside your collarbone and then in concentric circles inward on your breast until you reach the nipple. Check the nipple for cracks or oozing or inversion (the nipple sticking inside the areola).

Most people do not have symmetrical breasts, and many have irregularities that are totally normal. But if you feel a small, hard, pea-shaped lump under the surface, or if you're in doubt about any aspect of your exam, call your doctor at once.

All About Skin

A woman's skin is often her most prized possession—its softness, smoothness, and that proverbial "glow" may be one of her most attractive features. At this time of life, wrinkles may be a problem for some, but there are a variety of methods of caring for skin as you age.

Q: What makes wrinkles?
Skin is partly made of a protein called collagen, which responds to estrogen receptors all over the body. As we age, the process of skin cell replacement slows considerably, and the skin itself isn't as elastic as it used to be. The layer of fat cells under the skin declines.

In the first five years after menopause, we lose up to 30 percent of skin collagen, and the process continues (although more slowly) until death. Certain ethnic groups have fewer problems with this—African-American women typically don't wrinkle as early as Caucasian women, and many Hungarian and other Slavic women tend to retain their beautiful skin well into their seventies and eighties.

The sun is the worst photoager of all—the ultraviolet rays toughen and dry your skin. Renounce sunbathing if you want to stay young looking. Certain medications, such as antibiotics, tranquilizers, antidepressants, oral diabetes drugs, and diuretics, make you more susceptible to burning.

Smoking also dries the skin and helps to create wrinkles—there's another good reason to cut out cigarettes.

It's important to take good care of your skin at this age. Moisturizer is a must, and be sure to get one with a sunscreen, which will protect you from skin cancers and can also help to prevent the appearance of brown aging spots.

Q: Is there any cream that will make wrinkles less noticeable?

There are so many products on the market, and most of them are hardly worth the fancy jars they come in. A lot has been written about alpha-hydroxyacids, which take off layers of dead cells, but the most effective "wrinkle cream" is Retin-A, marketed as tretinoin cream, which must be prescribed by a dermatologist. (An over-the-counter product, called Renova, contains a certain amount of tretinoin, though not as much as the prescription variety. The over-the-counter products usually contain too little to make a significant difference on your skin.)

Another tip is to drink at least eight to ten glasses of water daily. The body is about 60 percent water and thrives on replacement of its natural fluids.

All About Weight Gain

Weight is a preoccupation with many women and never more so than at this time of life when the body appears to be shifting and changing even when you don't consume more calories. There are strategies for healthy eating and exercising that will help you through this volatile time of life.

Q: Why have I been gaining weight if I'm not eating more than I used to?

Menopause itself does not cause weight gain, but most women do gain weight at this time, often because their metabolism slows down. Also, the foods you used to eat aren't necessarily the foods you need now—the body doesn't process nutrients as efficiently as it used to, and much of what you eat turns to fat and fibrous tissue instead of muscle.

Many women who don't actually gain weight still complain that they look heavier because of a reapportionment of those pounds in undesirable places.

Q: Dieting used to work for me, and now it just makes me angry. What's a better solution to my weight problem?

Diets never work! It's never healthy to use drastic measures to get thin. A sensible eating program that includes all the major food groups and smaller portions is usually the answer. Reduce your intake of red meats, dairy products, and processed foods, and increase your consumption of fresh vegetables, fruits, grains, and legumes.

The best way to take weight off and keep it off is to exercise daily. You need at least twenty minutes a day of some aerobic activity—brisk walking, biking, rowing, step-training, racquet sports, dancing, martial arts, swimming, or hiking. And it's a good idea to cross-train, selecting an activity that will also give you endurance and strength, like tai chi or yoga.

Finally, although there are reports that HRT makes certain women gain weight, and that you reach more frequent plateaus when you're trying to lose weight, the fact of the matter is that many women do lose lean muscle mass and gain fat at menopause regardless of whether they take hormones. A good diet and an exercise program are vital in terms of weight management.

Q: Is it true that you're supposed to weigh a little more as you age?

Yes. At this time of life, an adrenal hormone called androstenedione is converted by the body's fat cells into estrone, a weaker form of estrogen. So the more fat cells you have, the more estrone is available to take care of other menopausal complaints. Putting on a few pounds if you're underweight also provides a little more padding for your bones and may protect you from fracture if you should fall.

Other Signs and Signals of Menopause

There are dozens of other signs and signals of menopause, from headaches to sore heels to ringing in the ears. If they bother you (and they may not), you can do something about them. All the menopausal possibilities listed below can be handled with appropriate techniques and treatments.

Q: I seem to get migraines all the time now. Why do they occur?

A migraine involves an imbalance in brain chemistry, the blood vessels in the scalp, and neurological messages that transmit pain. It is a one-sided headache, and often involves the whole body—other symptoms are light sensitivity, nausea, vomiting, and dizziness.

Migraines can be triggered by estrogen levels that are too low *or* too high, and can also be set off by hormone medications used to treat fibroids or endometriosis. Since estrogen encourages the production of beta endorphins, the natural opiates that alleviate pain, we have less resistance to the pounding of a migraine after menopause when our estrogen levels are low.

Q: What can I do about migraines?

One of the advantages of a classic migraine is that you usually get a warning—an aura such as a visible flash of light or a feeling that something is about to happen. This means you have time to set some preventive or reductive measures in motion. There are a variety of options, some of which may work sometimes—probably none of which will work all the time.

Discontinue HRT or work with your physician to reduce the amount of estrogen: A "natural" estrogen (see Chapter 7 for a description) may be tolerated better, as may a patch rather than a pill.

Try preventive medicine: Taking very low daily doses of a beta blocker or calcium channel blocker or a low-dose antidepressant or serotonin reuptake inhibitor may work for some women. However, these medications may all cause side effects. Imitrex (sumatriptan), which seemed to hold great promise for migraines, has been linked to heart attacks in people with no previous cardiac history. If you have had any chest pain while taking this medication, talk to your physician about discontinuing it.

Adjust your diet: A no-dairy, no-wheat diet seems to be very effective for some women. You should also strictly avoid red wine, aged cheese, chocolate, citrus fruits, nuts, and any food with additives or preservatives.

Enjoy a sexual romp: Although the migraine is the classic reason most women say, "Not tonight, darling," anecdotal evidence shows that getting aroused right at the moment that you feel the aura begin can redirect blood flow from the head to the genitals and also balance neurotransmitter production in the brain that will alleviate the pain.

Herbal solutions: Feverfew is the herb of choice for this problem. It inhibits the release of serotonin and also lowers prostaglandin levels (those hormones that sensitize the nervous system to pain). This herb must be taken daily, 15 to 20 drops of tincture. You may also wish to try tincture of vervain, black cohosh, or willow leaves. Peppermint oil and Chinese Tiger Balm can also be rubbed into your temples for topical relief.

Supplementation can help: Try vitamin B_6 (100 to 200 mg) daily, and be sure to take calcium and magnesium (1,200 and 600 mg, respectively); both have a calming effect on the nervous system and can balance neurotransmitter production. Some women have success with omega-3 fish oils. You should not take evening primrose or borage oil, which both contain prostaglandins.

Q: Why do my eyes feel so dry all the time?

All the body's mucous membranes—from the vagina to the mouth to the eyes—respond most fully under the influence of estrogen, so when we have less estrogen, we are effectively drier than we used to be. The eye, however, ages at its own rate, and estrogen is not the only factor—women on HRT don't necessarily have a better film of tears on the eye than those who don't take hormones.

Q: What can I do about dry eyes?

There are many helpful tactics you can use:

Exercise your eyes: Make sure you blink often. If you have a job where you stare at a computer screen all day, be sure to look around every few minutes.

Wash your eyes: Take a warm washcloth and press it to your lids until cool, then dip again in warm water. You can also wash your lids and eyelashes with a little diluted baby shampoo. Do this a couple of times a week to open the tear duct glands.

Stop smoking and stay out of smoke-filled rooms: Smoke dries the eye drastically.

Use liquid tears: There are a variety of products available in drugstores. Select the brands without preservatives and use three times daily or as needed.

Watch what you eat and drink: As with other menopausal problems, caffeine and alcohol dehydrate the cells; excess salt and sugar may interfere with gland secretions. Drink eight to ten glasses of water a day to replenish fluids.

Q: Why do I have a burning, dry mouth?

There are many reasons, but one is that as we lose estrogen, the mucosa in the mouth, which used to stay moist, no longer do. We may produce less saliva, which can exacerbate the problem.

Some other reasons may be hypersensitivities to food or

decayed matter left between the teeth, mouth ulcers or infections, and side effects of common medications.

To eliminate this problem, you must first have a dental checkup and take care of any infection that may be present. Next, you may wish to eliminate hot, spicy foods and increase your water intake. Ask your dentist whether using saliva substitutes might be advisable.

Q: Is it normal to feel tired all the time?

Fatigue is common to many menopausal women, but whether it's the result of night sweats disturbing sleep, poor living habits, or the attitude that many women seem to have that they must accomplish a hundred different things at the same time is unclear. You may need more sleep than usual while your hormones are in flux—treat yourself to an earlier bedtime and see if it helps.

Make sure you get out and exercise. Believe it or not, you can feel exhausted from not having the proper stimulation. A good workout also helps you sleep better.

Fatigue can also be a symptom of depression. If you can't get yourself out of bed in the morning, and nothing seems worth the effort, you should consult a professional and consider some short-term therapy.

Q: Is it strange that I sometimes hear ringing in my ears and that foods I used to love taste weird?

Sensory changes are often reported by menopausal women, and no one really knows why. The best thing you can do is try to calm down—meditate or listen to tapes of natural sounds. You may want to eat blander foods for a while, and then add back spices slowly, as you become accustomed to them again.

Q: I can't imagine why my heels and thumbs feel sore sometimes. Is there a reason for this?

Extremities often feel colder and get less circulation;

joints are also compromised with the loss of estrogen. Talk to your physician about whether she thinks that HRT might help to alleviate menopausal aching joints. At the same time, you might want to consider yoga or tai chi classes to return elasticity to older joints.

Q: Why can't I remember where I put the car keys or whether I took out the garbage? Am I losing my mind?

Memory loss is one of the most frightening of all menopausal symptoms, and it unfortunately is the one that has spawned generations of bad jokes and family ribbing about menopause that go, "Pay no attention to Mom. It's just her time to go nuts."

Why do we lose memory along with estrogen? In our reproductive years, this hormone causes plasticity of the synapses and dendrites in the nervous system and allows rapid, effective neurotransmission. So with the decline in hormones at menopause, it's quite common to lose some short-term memory, although nearly all women still operate within the range of normal. (Memory usually returns intact as the climacteric winds down.) It has been shown that HRT makes some difference—women who were on the medication had slightly better short-term verbal memory and better ability to learn new material. However, they scored no better than their nonmedicated sisters on general attention or visual-spatial memory.

Right now, it's a good idea to keep a notebook with you to jot down information you think you'll need quickly. Use visual cues (parking next to a bush cut in a certain configuration, for example, so you can remember where you put the car), or tape-record a list of things you have to do tomorrow and play them to yourself when you get up.

Q: How do I convince my physician that these signs and signals exist and that I'm not just a middle-aged hypochondriac?

If your doctor has a negative attitude, it's not your problem! You need a physician who is experienced in the treatment of menopausal women and has read the literature on all these symptoms. More important, you need someone who is sympathetic to your complaints and is willing to work with you—whether you choose hormones or natural therapies or both—to resolve your problems.

Chapter Four

Your Bones and Your Heart: The Real Reason for Estrogen Therapy

There are two serious health issues to consider at menopause that will emphatically affect your quality of life as you age and may also affect your longevity: your skeletal structure and changes in your heart and circulatory system.

Due to the diminished supply of estrogen in your body, your bones are no longer able to retain the same mass and density they had during your reproductive years, which leaves them susceptible to possible fracture and painful collapse.

The lack of estrogen in your bloodstream also alters the production of lipids or blood fats. This means that your cholesterol profile may change drastically over the next few years.

If you've had close family members who had osteoporosis or heart disease, you must be doubly concerned about your future. You must also be aware of your own personal risks when making the decision about taking HRT.

Even if you do choose to take medication, that's certainly not the complete answer. Nutrition, vitamin and mineral supplementation, exercise, and stress management are equally important in your health profile.

If you are active every day, that's a plus for your bones. And exercise will encourage you to stick with a low-fat diet, which is a plus for your heart. Adding fiber will not only keep your gastrointestinal system regular (and it often gets off track at menopause), but also enhances the cholesterol-lowering effect of a low-fat diet. And various supplements—calcium and magnesium for your bones, potassium and chromium for your heart—repair and restore the body in various excellent ways.

You can protect yourself from a heart attack and osteoporosis. Learning your risks, understanding the treatments, you will be able to make a wise choice now so that you can stay healthy for years to come.

All About Your Bones

The skeleton is the house we live in. It is built solidly to last for more than one hundred years. However, many elements conspire to erode the bones and make them thin and fragile. If we intend to be walking around on our hundredth birthday, we have to take care of our bones now.

Learning About Osteoporosis

This disease is a deadly and often silent illness—those who have it commonly don't know until a great deal of damage is already done. But armed with the right preventive tactics at fifty, you can help ensure that your bones will be in good shape at eighty or one hundred.

Q: What is osteoporosis?
Osteoporosis is a disease of imbalance that occurs when the amount of breakdown in bone tissue exceeds the

amount of buildup of new bone. The word means "porous bones," and the implications are wide ranging. This is a chronic disease that takes decades to manifest itself. As the years pass, the ratio of new bone to old bone shifts— the bone tissue of the skeleton is of good quality, but there's an insufficient quantity of it to support the body's activities.

Q: How does this degenerative process happen?
Bone is a dynamic tissue, always changing and remodeling itself. The skeleton you have today isn't the one you'll have ten years from now—each year, 10 percent of your bone turns over—but the older you are, the less new bone you get for the old bone that breaks down. In the osteoporotic process, the inside of the bone *(trabecular bone)* gets thinner while the outside *(cortical bone)* retains its shape. When the breakdown, or *resorption*, process happens faster than the buildup or remodeling process, the bone becomes osteoporotic.

Estrogen and other hormones in your body encourage the depositing of calcium into your bones, preventing it from leaching back into the bloodstream. But as your estrogen level declines at menopause, your bones can't hold on to the dietary calcium you take in and the endogenous calcium (calcium created by the body) you make. If the bone tissue gets too thin, it breaks easily— sometimes older women break a rib just by sneezing.

All women lose bone mass and density after menopause, because it takes estrogen to keep the calcium inside the bone tissue.

Q: How much bone could I safely lose without developing this disease?
If you're a normal bone loser (1 to 2 percent a year for the five to seven years following menopause), you may not have much to worry about. But if you're a fast loser (5 to 6

percent), you are at high risk for osteoporosis and are definitely a candidate for hormone replacement therapy.

Q: How would I suspect that I have osteoporosis?

You might not, if you didn't examine your risk factors. Osteoporosis works slowly and insidiously. There are usually no symptoms, although some women go through a rash of fractures at this time. Many women also notice that they are getting shorter. What's actually happening is that the disks of the spine are losing mass and compressing together, taking up less space than they used to.

When the density and mass of your bones reach a critical point, certain parts of your skeleton that are mostly composed of trabecular bone—the vertebrae, or the femoral neck of the hip, or the wrist—may begin to crumble. Osteoporotic bone doesn't heal well and often leaves the sufferer crippled. Vertebral breaks compress the spine and show up as the classic "dowager's hump," and hip fractures often leave an individual in a walker or wheelchair for life.

Q: What are my chances of getting osteoporosis?

More than twenty-five million Americans are currently affected by this disabling condition, which causes 1.3 million fractures a year in women and in some older, frail men. Osteoporosis attacks one-third to one-half of all postmenopausal women. Your lifetime risk of breaking a hip is greater than the *combined* risk of contracting breast, uterine, and ovarian cancer.

Risk Factors for Osteoporosis

If you know your risk factors, you'll be better able to make a judgment about HRT and other treatments. It's important to sort out the risks you can't change from those you can.

Q: What are the risk factors that I can't do anything about?

The first and most telling risk factor is age—the older you are, the greater your risk. The second is being female. Women have lighter, smaller bones to begin with, and because we go through menopause, we lose bone mass and density rapidly, within five to seven years after the last menstrual period. Petite women with small bones have an even greater risk. Men do get this disease, but typically, those most at risk are small and elderly.

Following this, you are at high risk if you have a family history of osteoporosis. If your mother and aunt had this condition, and your grandmother had a hump on her back and walked with a cane, you may be predisposed to develop the condition.

Your next factor is race—Caucasian women (particularly fair-haired and fair-skinned)—are the most likely to develop osteoporosis, and Asian-American women are next in line. Although African-American and Hispanic women do get this disease, it's not as common.

You are also more likely to develop osteoporosis if you've had your ovaries removed, since early surgical menopause means fewer years of estrogen in your body.

Q: Which are the risk factors I can change?

Lack of exercise is a big risk factor. If you don't get up and move your weight against gravity, your bones atrophy. Also, if you're sedentary, your muscles get out of practice supporting your weight, and you are more likely to fall awkwardly and sustain a break.

If you stop smoking, you can remove one big risk factor. Smokers tend to be thinner and go through menopause up to two years earlier than other women. Smoking also interferes with the formation of new bone tissue. Drinking alcohol is also detrimental to your bones—the ethanol creates more porous bones. High caffeine and soft drink consumption are also risk factors.

Another risk factor you may be able to do something about is bearing children. The pregnant body actually grows heavier bones as protection for the child inside, so if you've never had a child, you are at higher risk. A final risk factor is prolonged nursing without adequate restoration of calcium, which may deplete your body of calcium as you feed your child.

Diagnostic Testing for Osteoporosis

There are some excellent markers for bone to show how it has changed over time. We begin losing bone mass and density in our late thirties, and by fifty, it's important to know exactly how much of our skeleton is left. This can be a crucial factor in making the decision for or against HRT.

Q: Why would my doctor suggest that I have tests to determine my bone mass and density?

She might suggest tests if you have multiple risk factors for osteoporosis but are on the fence about taking HRT. She might also suggest these tests if you have recently suffered several fractures or are developing a hump on your back.

Q: What blood and urine tests should my doctor perform to check the mass and density of my bones?

Your doctor may suggest that you have biochemical (blood and urine) and radiological tests.

Blood tests will measure red and white blood cell counts, as well as protein, calcium, and hormone levels, and will show whether your bone turnover is more rapid than normal. Some tests will be performed to rule out other diseases of the bone. Urine tests will measure the difference between urinary calcium and creatinine, one of the nonprotein constituents of blood. If you are losing calcium rapidly over a twenty-four-hour period, your doctor will know you aren't absorbing sufficient calcium to help in the bone remodeling process.

Q: What radiological tests should my doctor perform?

Radiological tests, known as *bone densitometry testing*, are specialized X rays that measure your bone density. These tests can also be used as follow-ups after you've been on HRT for a year or so, to see how well you're responding to the therapy.

Bone mineral density shows up as a radiographic picture on a computer screen. While you lie on a table, a scanner checks your hips and spine, and the results come out as readings on a computer printout across the room. From these measurements, the machine age-matches you to normal women in their reproductive years and to women of your own age. The machine also estimates your fracture threshold—beneath the norm for your age, you are at risk; on the line or above it, you are within the norm for your age.

There are four types of measurements, all of which are noninvasive and painless and expose you to minimal doses of radiation:

Single-photon absorptiometry (SPA) passes photons from a radioactive source through your wrist or forearm and measures mass and density.

Dual-energy absorptiometry (DPA) is more precise. It uses beams from two radioactive sources and can examine thicker bone in the spine and hip. It measures both cortical and trabecular bone.

Dual-energy X-ray absorptiometry (DEXA) is the state-of-the-art diagnostic tool and uses an X-ray source rather than a radioisotope. It is more accurate, takes less time, and gives the patient a much lower dosage of radiation. The machine can examine hip, spine, and wrist.

Quantitative computed tomography (QCT) is a CT scanner with specialized software. This method costs the most, takes the longest time, and exposes you to higher doses of radiation. It is used to measure trabecular bone in the lower spine.

Q: What is a T-score, and how can I interpret whether or not it means I may have osteoporosis?

The T-score is the number of standard deviations below normal when compared to the measurement of a thirty-five-year-old woman. A score of 0 is average for a fifty- to fifty-five-year-old woman; a −1 is low-normal; a score of −2.5 is equivalent to a diagnosis of osteoporosis.

Q: How much do these tests cost, and will my insurance pay for them?

In most parts of the country, a hip and spine measurement costs about $300, and currently very few insurance companies will reimburse you. However, like mammograms, they are important tools for diagnosis, and if you are in a high-risk category, or if you and your doctor are at odds about whether you should be taking hormone replacement therapy, the cost may be worth it to you.

HRT and Osteoporosis

The best reason to take HRT is to protect your bones as you age by enabling you to retain good bone mass and density. Studies indicate that there is nothing else as effective. The only FDA sanction for hormone replacement therapy so far is for the prevention of osteoporosis.

Q: How does estrogen affect bone tissue?

Estrogen performs certain invaluable functions in the bone remodeling process. First, it inhibits bone resorption. During remodeling, cells called osteoclasts eat bone away, and other cells called osteoblasts build new bone. Estrogen helps to slow the breakdown—or resorption—process.

Then, too, there are special estrogen receptor sites—something like a keyhole for which estrogen is the key—in the osteoblasts. This means that each bone cell has a particular affinity for this hormone.

There may also be an insulin-like growth factor that helps estrogen work on the osteoblasts. And one final theory is that estrogen and a form of vitamin D found in the body may stimulate production of calcitonin, one of the hormones involved in the maintenance of bone mass.

Q: How does progesterone affect bone tissue?

There are progesterone receptors in bone, but they only appear in the presence of estrogen. One theory is that bone tissue accepts progesterone or progestin as an additional boost of estrogen, since progesterone breaks down to look like estrogen chemically once inside the body. There have been some studies that show that progesterone alone can build bone.

Q: What would HRT do for my bones?

Taking supplemental hormones will inhibit the resorption of bone and thus slow your loss. If you're a young woman with a small amount of bone loss, it is unlikely that you will *restore* any significant amount of bone mass and density with this medication. However, some elderly women with advanced osteoporosis have shown slightly higher bone density on tests after a year or so of medication.

Some studies show that HRT lowers the rate of hip fracture risk by 60 percent.

Q: How long would I have to take HRT to protect my bones?

Most experts have felt that you should start HRT no more than three years after your menopause and continue indefinitely. But if you live a very long life, this could mean thirty or forty years of exposure to hormone stimulation—and that could seriously compromise your breast cancer profile.

If you stop your course of medication, unfortunately, you will lose all the benefit you have gained while on it. That means that timing is everything—some physicians want you to start at menopause if you're losing bone quickly to slow the rate before you've lost too much. Others feel it's better to start later in life so that you can go longer. You'll have to discuss this with your own physician.

One new theory of administering HRT for osteoporosis is that unless you are a fast bone loser (determined by a bone absorptiometry test), it may be more prudent to wait to take medication until you're sixty-five or so, when your risk for osteoporosis is greater. The benefits of taking HRT in later life may be much more significant than taking it in midlife.

If you're a slow bone loser at fifty-five, with a T-score of 0, you would be advised to start right away only if you have multiple risk factors such as family history, heavy smoking and drinking, or fractures that won't heal. But if you are at -2 as you reach menopause, you should start immediately.

Q: My mother is seventy and has just been diagnosed with osteoporosis. Is it too late for her to start HRT?

Probably not, although there aren't many studies on HRT and advanced old age. Taking estrogen will slow bone loss no matter how old you are. However, most physicians feel that sixty-five or seventy is about as late as you can start to help retain what you've got and prevent enough loss to guard against broken hips or collapsed vertebrae.

Other Medications for Osteoporosis

Some women refuse hormones, and some can't take them. But there are drug prospects on the horizon that may be just as beneficial to your bones.

Q: Suppose I can't or don't want to take HRT. Are there any other drugs that are used for osteoporosis treatment?

There are, but they are usually only recommended for patients who have already been diagnosed with osteoporosis. Most of these drugs are still judged experimental, and some are not yet FDA approved for osteoporosis, although they are approved for other diseases of bone.

Calcitonin is derived from a hormone produced by a salmon that is very close to the human calcitonin, a hormone that blocks bone resorption. The hormone is inactivated by stomach acid, so you must either take it as an injection (daily, every other day, or three times a week, depending on your condition), or as a nasal spray.

Bisphosphonates are a category of drug that inhibits bone resorption by slowing down the action of the osteoclasts. The most commonly used member of this family has been Didronel (etidronate), which has had mixed results in clinical trials. It is also difficult to take, since the medication is cyclic and you have to chart your dosage carefully—you must be on it for two weeks out of every three months. A newer bisphosphonate is Fosamax (alendronate). It has only just finished its clinical trials and hit the commercial market, and experts feel that it has several advantages over its cousin Didronel, including ease of administration (you take a small daily dose). It is also safer to take since the medication doesn't stay in the bone as long as Didronel. However, it's really too soon to judge how effective it will be.

Slow-release sodium fluoride has been popular in Europe for years, although it is rarely prescribed in the United States. It was found that fluoride did create new bone, but it wasn't strong and new breaks occurred easily. However, the jury is still out on the efficacy of this treatment—research facilities are experimenting with lower dosages than were previously used.

Natural Treatments to Protect Your Bones

If you decide that you do not wish to take any medication, or if you cannot take drugs because of a conflicting medical condition, there are plenty of natural remedies that may help.

Q: What natural treatments are available for osteoporosis and how effective are they?

You have a wide range, from calcium supplementation, diet, and exercise to herbal therapy. None of these has been shown to equal the dramatic results of HRT on bone mass and density. However, a combination of natural treatments will keep your bones healthy and make your entire body more resilient. In working holistically, from the inside out, you will be taking care of all systems of your body, including those cells and tissues that support the skeleton and limbs.

Q: What will taking dietary and supplemental calcium do for my bones?

Calcium plays a very important part in the architecture of the skeleton. Bone takes up about 99 percent of the calcium in our bodies—the rest of the available calcium we have, which is carried in the blood, is used in nerve transmission, blood clotting, and muscle contraction.

In order to expedite the remodeling process of the bones, we need a balanced flow of calcium passing back and forth between the blood and bones. Certain bone cells have estrogen receptor sites, like gates that open when estrogen is present, to inhibit the breakdown process. When we reach menopause, and the number of receptor sites declines along with the estrogen, we have an increased need for more dietary calcium. Women in their seventies and eighties have an even greater need for calcium, since as we age, it's much harder to absorb and utilize the calcium we get from food.

Q: What foods should I eat that are rich in calcium?
Most people think of dairy products as good calcium sources, and they are—just make sure you consume low-fat or reduced-fat dairy. You can get plenty of calcium from the following sources:

Green Leafy Vegetables
(1-cup serving, cooked)

rhubarb (stem only)	348 mg calcium
collard greens	300
spinach	278
turnip greens	229
bok choy	200
kale	179
broccoli	150

Sea Vegetables
(1-cup serving, cooked; available in Asian markets)

hijiki	610
dulse	567
wakame	520

Fish with Bones

salmon, 1 cup canned	431
sardines, 3^1/$_2$-oz. can	300

Beans and Legumes

tempeh, 4 oz.	172
chickpeas, 1 cup	150
black beans, 1 cup	135
pinto beans, 1 cup	128

Nuts and Seeds

almonds, 1 cup	300
hazelnuts, 1 cup	282
sunflower seeds, 1 cup	174

Dairy

skim milk, 1 cup	300
cheese (American, Swiss, 1^1/$_2$ oz.)	300
nonfat yogurt, 1 cup	294
whole milk, 1 cup	288
ice milk, 1 cup	204

You should also cut down on processed foods, high-phosphate sodas, alcohol, and caffeine. All of these cause a greater excretion of urinary calcium.

Q: How much supplemental calcium should I take?

Very few women eat enough calcium-rich foods to affect their bones. Even if your diet is heavy in calcium, your gut doesn't absorb nutrients the way it did when you were younger. For this reason, you should supplement over and above what you are eating. If you are not taking HRT, you should be taking 1,000 to 1,200 mg of calcium daily if you're pre- or perimenopausal, 1,500 mg of calcium daily if you're postmenopausal. If you are taking HRT, you should still take 1,000 mg of calcium daily.

The most available form of calcium (the one your digestive system can break down most easily so that this supplement is quickly absorbed into your bloodstream) is calcium citrate. You may also take calcium carbonate or a blend of the two. Calcium should be taken with food for the best absorption.

Q: Why do I need to take magnesium with calcium?

Magnesium makes the calcium more available to the bones. It also helps the body to use vitamin D and to maintain bone integrity.

Q: What foods contain magnesium?

You can get this mineral in millet, potatoes, corn, wheat, brown rice, barley, and lentils. Unfortunately, cooking washes away a lot of the nutrient value, which means that you should be supplementing magnesium as well.

Q: How much supplemental magnesium should I take?

The usual amount is about half of the calcium you're taking. Some health food stores carry a formula which gives calcium, magnesium, plus boron, a trace mineral that also helps to get the calcium working better in the body.

Q: Will vitamin D help my bones?

Yes, but you don't need to supplement it in your diet if you get out into the sunlight at least once a day. In the winter, in the northern states, it's a good idea to eat fish or take fish-oil supplements as well as take a walk in the fresh air to be sure you have enough D.

Q: Are there any other minerals I should take to improve my bone density?

You should have 1,000 mg of phosphorus daily; 2 grams of sodium or less, and about 5 to 7 grams of potassium (unless you have kidney problems, in which case your potassium should be as low as possible).

As for micronutrients (those you don't have to supplement, but which should be included in your daily diet), you need a good mix of selenium (often packaged with vitamin E), chromium, copper, boron, silicon, zinc, cobalt, and sulfur. These are essential for bone strength and flexibility. You can find these micronutrients in seaweeds such as wakame, nori, or kelp.

Q: What's the best exercise for my bones?

Any activity that moves your body against gravity is great. This includes walking, jogging, biking, rowing, racket sports, dancing, yoga, low-impact aerobics, hiking, martial arts, or weight training. Swimming, although wonderful for your body, is not particularly beneficial for your bones, since your weight is supported by the water.

Studies have shown that gait and balance are crucial in the prevention of falls and fractures. As we age, we often lose the surefootedness we used to have, and may slip on uneven pavement or accidentally stumble down a stair. The best exercise to restore balance is tai chi chuan, which teaches mind and body how to move in space. (See Chapter 3 for a description of this Chinese meditative art.)

The important thing about exercise is that you should be doing something every day. If you get up half an hour earlier in the morning, do some stretches, and take a brisk walk, you are making a big contribution to your bone health.

Q: Are there any herbs that will strengthen my bones?

The two traditional herbs used are comfrey, also called "knitbone," and horsetail, which thickens and stabilizes bone tissue. You can drink infusions of this, or sit in a bathtub to which you have added a few cups of horsetail-comfrey tea.

You can also take nettle or dandelion (10 to 15 drops tincture in a glass of water) about fifteen minutes before you eat.

Q: What commonsense measures should I use to protect my bones at midlife?

This is an ideal time to safety-proof your environment. Wear flats instead of heels and give away your floor-length skirts, coats, and bathrobes. If you need eyeglasses or contacts, wear them, and if things still look blurry, make an appointment for an eye exam. If your doctor has recommended that you use a cane, do so.

This is a good time to reevaluate your medications. If you feel woozy a good deal of the time, perhaps you are combining drugs inappropriately or taking too much of a certain drug. (The same advice goes for alcohol—a glass of wine with dinner is fine and may even strengthen your bones and heart, but overindulging will destroy your balance and make you prone to falls.)

Be careful lifting, bending, stooping, or shoveling. If you can get someone else to do heavy labor for you—even opening a stuck window—do so. Look around your house and outside it for possible danger zones. Tack down electrical wires, fix broken sidewalks, and watch out for dogs and cats underfoot. Be sure to keep a night-light near your bed and one in the bathroom, should you have to get up at night.

All About Your Heart

Learning About Female Heart Disease

The heart, that great muscular pump, keeps us going day and night throughout our life span. It can, however, be damaged or become dysfunctional from a variety of causes. At menopause, with the loss of estrogen, the heart becomes more susceptible to disease. When we learn more about this organ and the circulatory system that supports it, it is easier to understand what we can do to protect it.

Q: Why is the female heart different from the male heart?

Women's hearts are smaller than men's and beat more often and more quickly both at rest and in motion. Our coronary arteries (the arteries that feed the heart muscle itself) are also smaller—this means that they may close up more quickly when occluded with plaque, and that they are harder to work on surgically.

Women's hearts are protected throughout their reproductive years by the abundance of estrogen they produce (men only have a little in their system), which has a beneficial effect on lipids. Estrogen keeps HDL cholesterol (the good cholesterol) high and LDL (the bad cholesterol) low.

The female heart reacts differently than the male heart to physical and emotional stress. When a woman is put on a treadmill and asked to walk against resistance, an electrocardiograph reading may show patterns that can be interpreted as abnormal even though they're not.

Q: Why is women's heart disease different from male heart disease?

Women's heart disease develops about ten years after men's, when the protective effects of estrogen are no longer available to the heart and circulatory system.

The common pattern for male heart disease is that the

first symptom is a heart attack. If the man survives this catastrophic event, he will undoubtedly be recommended for an angioplasty, where a small balloon is inserted into the coronary arteries and expanded to smash the plaque up against the artery walls and open the passageway, or a bypass, where a vein from the leg or chest is used to divert blood flow from the blocked artery. He is more likely to be recommended for physical therapy after his procedure and to be closely monitored by physicians and therapists through recovery.

The common pattern for female heart disease is often a long history of chest pain (angina) and shortness of breath, which may be dismissed by the woman as indigestion or the aches and pains of aging. Another typical pattern is that the woman has no symptoms at all and simply collapses from a heart attack without warning. Women are rarely recommended for the types of diagnostic cardiac tests that men get during a routine physical in midlife. By the time a woman is seen by a cardiologist, she is usually older and sicker, and may be a poor candidate for surgery.

Q: What are my chances of developing heart disease?
More than 250,000 American women a year die of heart attacks, and if you count deaths from all coronary artery and blood vessel diseases, the total is 500,000 women's lives each year. You are six times as likely to die of heart disease than breast cancer and twice as likely to die of a stroke than lung cancer.

Q: With numbers so large, why is women's heart disease not at the top of the news?
One-third of women's heart attacks go unreported, either because they are "silent" (without any symptoms), or because women deny that anything is wrong. Many women suffer years of pain and are unaware of how much

damage has been done. Also, many doctors still refuse to believe that coronary artery disease is a woman's problem. They are much more likely to attribute the chest pain and shortness of breath to indigestion or "aches and pains of aging."

What Can Go Wrong with Your Heart? Symptoms and Conditions

It's important to understand the various problems to which the heart is susceptible. When you are more knowledgeable about the different types of heart disease, you will be better able to explain your symptoms and complaints to your physician.

Q: What are the symptoms of women's heart disease?
You may feel any of the following symptoms singly or together. If you experience any of these symptoms on a regular basis, *see your doctor at once*:

- chest pain (especially midchest)
- palpitations (pounding of the heart), bumping, fluttering, or flopping
- blackouts or fainting
- shortness of breath
- great fatigue

Q: Is every chest pain I have angina? What does angina really feel like?
You may have pain in your chest from hiatal hernias, gallbladder disease, or anxiety. But if you feel a pain right in the middle of your chest that is *crushing, constricting, aching, squeezing, burning, strangling, like indigestion, like an elephant sitting on your chest, like a heavy pressure, tight, cold, heavy, clammy,* or *full*, that is angina.

Q: Why should menopause put me at higher risk for cardiovascular disease?

Heart attacks, atherosclerosis, and other cardiac diseases rarely occur in women of reproductive age because of high estrogen levels that keep blood lipids (HDLs and LDLs) in balance. But after menopause, when levels drop to within 20 percent of what they used to be, we lose the protective effects on our heart. (See below for a description of the effects of HRT on the heart.)

Q: Which cardiac conditions might I be susceptible to?

The most common forms of heart disease that afflict women are:

Atherosclerosis: This disease is caused by the formation of fatty deposits known as plaques on the walls of the coronary arteries. When the plaques are very large, they can block blood supply, and it becomes increasingly difficult for the heart to receive the blood it needs to function. Angina—crushing chest pain—is a typical symptom of atherosclerosis. If the arteries are completely blocked, cutting off the oxygen supply to the heart, a heart attack can result.

Silent ischemia: Ischemia is a deficiency in the oxygen supply to the heart. In women, it is often common for this to occur without any pain whatsoever. The damage to the heart may occur and not be detected until much later, when it shows up on an electrocardiogram (EKG).

Hypertension: When the blood is forced to travel through the arteries at high pressure, the heart has to work harder and uses more oxygen to do this work. High pressure in the arteries can damage arterial walls and cause a buildup of plaque, which can develop into atherosclerosis.

Syndrome X: This condition, which is almost unique to women, occurs in healthy individuals who occasionally have acute attacks of anginal pain. The problem appears to be microscopic, happening at a cellular level too small to detect in regular diagnostic tests. HRT has been found to be extremely effective in treating syndrome X.

Stroke: When blood flow cannot reach the brain, many brain cells are killed off or irreparably damaged, resulting in impairment of movement, vision, speech, or memory. Strokes may be caused by blockages on artery walls leading from the heart to the brain, by ruptured blood vessels, or by blood clots that occur elsewhere in the body and travel to the brain.

Cardiac arrhythmias: Arrhythmias are problems with the electrical functioning of the heart. When the chambers of the heart contract in nonrhythmic or atypical beats, they can prevent blood flow from the heart from getting to the rest of the body. *Fibrillation* (abnormal contraction) may occur in the upper heart chambers (the *atria*) or, more seriously, in the lower chambers (the *ventricles*), where it can result in death.

Pericarditis: This condition, an inflammation of the sac that surrounds the heart, brings on pain when you breathe or change position. It is often triggered by a viral infection, or may be a secondary problem after a heart attack.

Mitral valve prolapse: This congenital condition (a condition that occurs at birth) is usually not serious, and most commonly occurs in women. In a normal heart, the valve that separates the upper from the lower chambers closes tight after blood has passed through. But in mitral valve prolapse, the valve is enlarged and "floppy," allowing some blood to seep back into the atrium. This can result in chest pain (unlike angina, it is usually intermittent, and on the left side), dizziness, numbness, and panicky or anxious feelings. Arrhythmias may also occur.

Risk Factors for Heart Disease

All of us have many risks, some of which are controllable, and some of which simply come with the territory of being a woman past menopause. But if you are diligent about taking care of the risk factors you *can* alter, you may be able to beat the odds on the ones that you can't change.

Q: Which risk factors for heart disease are out of my control?

Age and gender both put you at risk. When you are a woman past menopause, you no longer enjoy the protective effects of estrogen on your heart.

Your family history is a considerable risk factor. If you have one or more immediate family members who had a heart attack or heart disease under the age of fifty-five, you are at higher risk yourself.

Your race may put you at higher risk—African-American, Hispanic, and women from certain Native American tribes are more at risk than Caucasians.

Q: Which risk factors are under my control?

Your cholesterol levels can be managed with diet, exercise, and medication if necessary. HDLs should be higher than 45, LDLs lower than 130; total less than 200.

Your triglyceride levels are an independent risk factor because you are a woman. Triglycerides should be kept below 130.

Your blood pressure should be under 140/90 to be at normal risk.

Diabetes is a risk factor you can't control. However, you can manage your disease and be sure that your cholesterol, blood glucose, and blood pressure are kept under control.

If you're obese, this is a considerable risk that you can alter in a weight-reduction program. You should be no more than 20 percent above life insurance tables norms.

Stress can elevate blood pressure and cause cardiac arrhythmias. Women are at high risk if they feel harried and overwhelmed most of the time.

Smoking, and particularly smoking in combination with taking birth control pills, is a risk factor. Smoking can lead to blood clots and constricted blood vessels; the levels of estrogen and progestin in the Pill (five times higher than that in HRT) can accentuate the body's propensity for blood clots.

Alcohol in moderation (one glass of wine a day) is good for your heart; but drinking to excess fills the body with toxins the heart and liver cannot process adequately.

Poverty and social isolation are risk factors as well. Elderly women who can't afford medical care and live on their own have a higher-than-average chance of succumbing to heart disease.

Diagnostic Testing for Heart Disease

You need a good picture of your heart at midlife, a clearer one than is offered by a simple blood pressure and heart rate check. The diagnostic tests available will give your physician a good idea of what shape your heart is in now, and what to expect in the future.

Q: What tests might my doctor do to find out whether I'm at risk for heart disease?

If you're a woman past fifty, it's a good idea to have basic cardiac testing in your general wellness exam the next time you see your physician. If you're younger, but your blood pressure is consistently high, if you have chest pain or shortness of breath, or if you have a strong family history of heart disease, you should certainly have one or several of the following tests:

Routine blood and urine tests: Urine tests will let you know whether you're spilling sugar into your urine (indicating diabetes) or red blood cells (which might indicate kidney damage). Blood tests will check HDL and LDL levels, triglycerides, and thyroid hormone levels.

EKG (electrocardiogram): This test will show abnormalities in the electrical activity of the heart, arrhythmias, and sometimes signs of ischemia (deficiency of blood supply to the heart).

Exercise stress testing (with thallium): You will be asked to walk against increasing resistance on a treadmill as your heart rate and blood pressure are checked and a baseline EKG is taken. Since women's hearts may show abnormalities even when there is no disease, a much more accurate test involves injecting a thallium (radioactive dye) tracer into your blood and watching its progress through the arteries on a screen as you walk the treadmill.

Echocardiogram: This ultrasound test shows the workings of your heart and its valves and the size of the chambers. It can also detect diseases of the heart muscles from hypertension.

Cardiac catheterization: During this test, a catheter is run from a vein in your groin or arm into the heart. A contrast dye is injected into the vein, and its progress through the circulatory system shows whether there are blockages in your arteries.

EPS (electrophysiology study): Similar to catheterization, this test determines the cause of arrhythmias by inserting a tube with pacemaker wires through a vein in your groin or arm into your heart.

Making a Decision About HRT for Heart Disease

Although HRT is still not FDA approved for the prevention of heart disease, it has been shown to be very effective in dozens of clinical trials. The evidence is very persuasive—women on HRT have a 40 to 50 percent reduction in heart disease as compared with nonusers. You and your physician may wish to discuss the possibilities of HRT if you are in a high-risk category.

Q: What does HRT do for the heart and circulatory system?

Estrogen serves several functions in premenopausal women to keep atherosclerotic plaque from adhering to arteries. The key appears to be that vascular smooth muscle cells contain estrogen receptors and therefore respond directly to estrogen exposure. Heart attacks are relatively rare in young women, undoubtedly due to the normally high estrogen levels that exist in reproductive-age women. Replacing estrogen after menopause will protect the smooth muscle cells in the same way.

Hormone replacement does not reduce the levels of another lipid, the triglycerides, and evidence from the PEPI trials (see page 80) shows that oral HRT may actually increase them. These lipids are naturally higher in women than in men, and can be an independent risk factor for heart disease.

Estrogen also gives better vascular elasticity. One theory of why women don't get heart attacks when they're pregnant, despite their increased blood volume and higher blood pressure, is that estrogen allows the blood vessels to expand to accommodate a bigger workload.

Finally, estrogen also protects women by reducing another form of LDL cholesterol known as LP(a), which when elevated after menopause can cause stroke.

Q: If I have a uterus and have to take progesterone as well as estrogen, will that help or hurt my heart?

Clinical trial results have been very confusing on this score. Apparently, the most protection you can get for your heart is ERT—taking unopposed estrogen. However, if you have a uterus, you must take a progestin or natural progesterone in order to be certain that the lining of the uterus (the endometrium) doesn't overgrow under the influence of estrogen.

The addition of a progestin means that you may not get

the full cardiovascular protection you get on ERT. The effects of progestin on cholesterol are not well understood, but we know that it does lower HDL levels. It also removes some good antioxidant benefits that you get from estrogen, which can be protective against cancer.

There's also some indication that you get better lipid profiles by taking HRT orally, and the combined continuous regimen (where you take your hormones daily) may be preferable to the cyclic regimen (where you take hormones for most of the month and then stop for several days) when thinking about cardiovascular benefits. (See Chapter 7 for a full description of these regimens.)

Some experts feel that when the dosage of estrogen is right for the particular woman, the addition of the progestin doesn't take away from its beneficial cardiovascular effects. Others feel that natural progesterone, which does not reduce HDL cholesterol, is the best solution for women with an intact uterus. You will have to discuss these options with your physician before making a decision.

If you have an intact uterus and dislike the progestin part of the drug regimen, you and your physician should discuss the advisability of skipping a month, or at the outside, skipping two months of the progestin. If you elect to do this, you should have a transvaginal ultrasound or an endometrial biopsy every six months to a year to ensure that your endometrium remains healthy.

Q: What kinds of clinical trial testing have been done to indicate that HRT is a good option for my heart?
The results of the Postmenopausal Estrogen and Progestin Interventions Trial (PEPI), a three-year study of nearly nine hundred women released in November 1994, showed that HRT has a beneficial impact on coronary risk factors. Some women were given a placebo, some took estrogen alone, and the remaining women were split between those who took estrogen plus a progestin and

those who took estrogen plus natural micronized progesterone. The most benefit (the greatest rise in HDL cholesterol) was seen in those taking estrogen alone; the next best results were seen in those taking the combination of estrogen plus natural progesterone. The natural product also caused fewer side effects than the synthetic.

Unfortunately, the questions about benefits and risks of long-term use have yet to be answered. The HRT arm of the Women's Health Initiative study will not be finished until 2005.

Q: Should I consider HRT if I've already been diagnosed with heart disease or have had a heart attack?

The best candidates for HRT, some doctors feel, are those who've already had a heart attack or have been diagnosed with coronary artery disease. You already know that you are at high risk, and you know you can improve your lipid profile with medication, which means that you can only live longer on HRT (or ERT if you have no uterus). Observational reports indicate that there is a 70 to 90 percent reduction in deaths for women with established heart disease who begin to take HRT.

When hormone replacement is used solely as a preventive measure in healthy women, the only apparent result is a reduction in cholesterol and triglycerides. But in proven heart disease, the medication also stabilizes lesions and enhances the functioning and elasticity of the blood vessels.

HRT is advisable for women with atherosclerosis, syndrome X, coronary artery stenosis (narrowing of the arteries), cardiac arrhythmias, mitral valve prolapse, and pericarditis. Be sure to discuss your risks and benefits with your physician.

If you have had a pulmonary embolism or deep vein thrombosis, it is questionable whether you should take

HRT. High estrogen levels in contraceptives often *cause* these cardiac problems, particularly in smokers, so it is not yet known whether the lower levels of estrogen in HRT are safe for someone with this type of medical history. Most physicians who do prescribe HRT for patients with embolisms or thrombosis use the transdermal patch, since it does not encourage the production of coagulation proteins in the liver as the pills do.

Q: What if I've had breast cancer? Should I take HRT to protect my heart anyway?

This is a very hard call, and it will take some time and serious discussion with your physician to make it. Any estrogen-dependent cancer is usually grounds for prohibiting replacement estrogen. And then, too, some studies indicate that the progestin may also increase your risk of breast cancer. (There is not enough data on breast cancer and either hormone to condemn both or either.)

The answer may be that you've already *had* breast cancer and therefore your risk of a recurrence is probably higher than your risk of getting heart disease. Many women also say that even though heart disease is the number one killer of American women, they are more concerned about dying of cancer. Only you can decide what your top health priority is. Discuss this thoroughly with your physician before making your decision.

Other Medications and Procedures for Heart Disease

If you have already been diagnosed with heart disease, there are a variety of medications and procedures that can help your condition, regardless of whether you choose to take HRT.

Q: What are the most commonly prescribed drugs to treat heart disease?

The most common drugs are nitroglycerin for angina; diuretics to reduce salt and water in the body and thereby help to lower blood pressure; beta blockers, which lower the heart's demand for oxygen under stress; and calcium channel blockers, which prevent spasms in coronary arteries by lowering the amount of calcium going into the muscle cells of the artery walls.

In addition, your doctor may prescribe cholesterol-lowering drugs, aspirin and other anticoagulants to thin your blood, vasodilators to open your blood vessels, and antiarrhythmia drugs to slow down or stop erratic heartbeats.

Q: If noninvasive diagnostic procedures and medication don't help, what other treatments are available?

The next step is to try and open the narrowed arteries, or bypass the blocked arteries.

Balloon angioplasty: In this procedure, a catheter with a small balloon on the end is passed through a vein from the groin or arm into the heart. The coronary arteries are visualized on a monitor and the catheter brought to the blockage, where the balloon is then inflated, pressing the plaque against the artery walls and stretching the narrowed opening so that blood can flow through it again.

Coronary bypass surgery: If angioplasty has failed to open the blockages, you may be a candidate for a bypass. A vein is taken from your leg or chest and grafted onto the diseased artery, creating a new avenue for your coronary blood supply.

Nonmedical Treatments to Protect Your Heart

You can't rely solely on medication and surgery to take good care of your heart. Whether you are concerned about staying in great cardiac shape as you age or you have already been diagnosed with heart disease, the following therapies will make your life and your heart stronger and healthier.

Q: Which alternative therapies will protect me against heart disease or help if I already have been diagnosed with heart disease?

There are many, including diet and exercise, vitamin and mineral and "quasi"-vitamin supplementation, herbs, homeopathy, and stress management techniques such as meditation, yoga, and tai chi.

Q: What should I eat for a preventive heart-healthy diet?

It's important that you design a diet you will stick to and that will be beneficial to your heart. The first maxim is keep the fat in your food as low as possible. Although the figure of 20 percent of daily calories from fat is the amount recommended by the U.S. Department of Health and Human Services, some experts feel that the only way to prevent heart disease or keep healthy after a heart attack is to reduce the fat in your diet to 10 to 15 percent.

You need a well-rounded menu plan that includes fresh fruits, vegetables, grains, cereals, and legumes (which offer plenty of vegetable protein), and just a little bit of animal protein from lean meat, poultry without skin, and fish. Dairy products should be cut to a minimum, and the products you do buy should be low-fat or reduced-fat.

You should have plenty of fiber and soy in your diet as well. (See chapter 10 for a description of enhancing the estrogen in your body by eating soy products.)

Q: What does fiber do for my heart?

Soluble fiber, the indigestible cell-wall material of plant cells, when added to a low-fat diet, reduces cholesterol dramatically. This type of fiber is found in oats and oat bran, fruits like apples, blackberries, peaches, pears, plums, and dried peas and beans. It can reduce LDLs by as much as 24 percent and total cholesterol by 26 percent in just twenty-four weeks. In one twelve-year study, this dramatic lowering of cholesterol levels resulted in a 25 percent reduction of deaths from coronary heart disease.

High-fiber diets also offer protection against diabetes and assist the body in maintaining good blood sugar levels and increasing its sensitivity to insulin (which helps to process fats and sugars efficiently).

Q: How much and what type of fiber should I eat?

You should eat from 25 to 35 grams of fiber daily—any more than that and you may be interfering with the body's ability to absorb calcium. Be sure you eat the skin on your potato and apple; buy cereal that has at least 3 grams of fiber per serving, and switch from white to whole-grain bread. You can also purchase cereal that contains the high-fiber psyllium seed (Uncle Sam's is one commonly available brand).

Add fiber to your diet slowly to give your body time to adapt. You will find that your gastrointestinal system is much more active than it used to be—and it's fine for you to eliminate more often as long as your stomach doesn't become upset.

Q: Is it vital for my heart to take vitamin and mineral supplements?

Yes. Even though you may eat an exemplary diet, the body absorbs fewer nutrients as you get older, and they are more readily available to the body in supplemental form. Vitamins, minerals, "quasi"-vitamins, enzymes, essential fatty acids, and amino acids all aid in the fight against aging and degenerative disease.

Q: Should I take a multivitamin? What should it contain?

Yes. At menopause it's important to have a multivitamin that includes the antioxidant vitamins A, C, and E with selenium; a whole range of B vitamins (B_1, B_2, B_6, B_{12}, niacin, and folate); and the minerals calcium, magnesium, zinc, chromium, potassium, and phosphorus. (See pages 67–68 for a full discussion of supplemental calcium and magnesium for bone strength.)

Niacin supplements, taken with meals three times daily, have been found to be protective against heart disease. However, they can cause a hot-flash–like flush and gastrointestinal problems. Discuss this supplement with your physician before taking it, and ask if you can reduce the dosage or discontinue use if you have side effects.

Q: I've heard that Coenzyme Q-10 is beneficial for the heart. What does it do?

Co-Q-10, also known as ubiquinone, is really a vitamin that helps to regulate the flow of oxygen in the cells. It is particularly good for the heart and is often used as a treatment for angina. Even in cases of serious cardiac disease, it improves heart function. It also has antioxidant properties and helps to spark cellular energy in the body.

The typical protective dose for healthy individuals is 10 to 20 mg daily for about six to twelve months, but if you have heart disease, you can safely take 120 to 360 mg daily.

Q: Which amino acids might help my heart?

Both lysine (500 mg daily on an empty stomach) and L-carnitine (500 to 1,000 mg daily) are helpful in cholesterol metabolism. Lysine makes one type of cholesterol less sticky so that it cannot adhere to arteries; carnitine affords better oxygen flow to blood cells, reduces triglyceride levels, and raises HDLs.

Q: Should I be taking essential fatty acids (EFAs)?

Many experts feel that EFAs are particularly beneficial for menopausal women because they stimulate the production of prostaglandins, hormonelike substances that participate in many different activities in the body. Prostaglandins help to reduce pain (they are an active ingredient in PMS-relief-type drugs). They also prevent blood platelets from clumping together and, in so doing, keep plaque off artery walls.

The particular type of fatty acid you should be taking is linoleic acid, which is converted by the body into GLA (gamma-linoleic acid). It is once again converted by an enzyme process into prostaglandins.

Q: I've heard that evening primrose oil is wonderful for your heart. What is it?

The evening primrose plant (one widely available brand is efamol) contains gamma-linoleic acid, so when you take it, your body gets GLA directly, without having to go through the conversion process.

The appropriate protective dosage is 500 mg three times daily. This oil has been known to alleviate hot flashes, fatigue, insomnia, and other menopausal complaints. It also lowers serum cholesterol and reduces the risk of thrombosis.

This is a highly estrogenic oil, and therefore if you are at risk for estrogen-dependent cancer, you should substitute borage oil or black currant oil, which also contain GLA.

Q: What are the benefits of the omega-3 fatty acid called EPA?

EPA (eicosapentaenoic acid), a fish oil, is also a precursor to prostaglandins. If you eat a lot of cold water fish, such as cod, mackerel, and herring, or take supplemental EPA (1,000 to 2,000 mg daily), you will be lowering your cholesterol levels and triglycerides, controlling arterial spasms, and preventing the production of blood clots.

Q: Are there any heart-healthy herbs I can take?
Yes, but if you are already on heart medication, you must be sure to inform your physician before taking herbs. The following herbs are compatible with hormone replacement therapy, but some should not be taken in combination with other heart drugs. You may take ½ to 1 teaspoon of the dried herb in a cup of boiling water twice daily, or a half-dropperful of extract in half a glass of water three times daily.

Hawthorn: which enhances cardiac output
Garlic: which blocks the biosynthesis of cholesterol
Yarrow: a diuretic to rid the body of excess fluid
Dandelion: a kidney tonic and diuretic
Burdock root: a blood cleanser
Ginkgobiloba: a vasodilator for the blood vessels in the brain.

Q: What homeopathic remedies are good for the heart?
Homeopathy uses small doses of elements that might be harmful in larger doses to encourage the body to raise its natural immune defenses. Some homeopathic remedies for heart problems are:

Aconitum napellus: for palpitations and fear of the onset of a heart attack. IF YOU ARE HAVING A HEART ATTACK, YOU MUST GET EMERGENCY CARE AT THE SAME TIME.
Apis: for fluid retention and swelling
Arnica: for a sore, bruised feeling, any physical trauma
Aurum metallicum: for hypertension and depression

Cactus: for disturbed blood flow, valve disease
Latrodectus mactans: for angina, pain midchest

Q: How much exercise do I need to protect my heart?

Physical activity not only reduces cholesterol levels and maintains a healthy weight; it also reduces stress. In order to be fit, you should be doing some form of aerobic activity every day, for twenty minutes a day, enough to get your heart up to its maximum rate and then, as you cool off, back to normal. A brisk two-mile walk every day will give you the level of fitness you need for a healthy heart.

But aerobics aren't enough. To get the total benefit for your heart, you also need endurance, strength, and flexibility, so it's a good idea to cross-train. Yoga and stretching will make you flexible; tai chi or swimming will give you endurance; weight training will make you strong.

If you have been diagnosed with heart disease, you must have your doctor's okay before you begin any exercise program. Studies have shown that physical therapy after a heart attack—where you are monitored on a variety of exercise machines for several months—provides the most complete recovery. Exercise also complements diet. You are more likely to stick to your good nutrition program when you feel and look fit.

Q: What does stress do to my heart?

When we are pressured or angry, our brain sends a message to the adrenal glands to start pumping out the "stress hormones," also known as the "fight or flight" hormones. When flooded with *adrenalin*, *noradrenalin*, and *cortisol*, our muscles tense and arteries constrict. This can lead to blood clots or spasms in blood vessels.

Q: What can I do to reduce my stress levels?

A regular program of meditation, breathing, yoga, or

tai chi will do a lot to reduce your stress. We all have various triggers for our anger and frustration, but we don't have to succumb to them. The first (and easiest) suggestion for stress management, when you are filled with rage at a bad driver, at a difficult boss, or at your spouse or child, for example, is to count to ten (and breathe deeply as you do so). You can also take a sitting break where you meditate quietly and focus on your breath or a word such as "Peace" or "Om." Try to schedule activities so that you never get overwhelmed with obligations—block in some time for relaxation each day. You deserve a break, and so does your heart.

Chapter Five

Is Estrogen Safe?

If only taking estrogen were like eating the proverbial apple every day. It would be safe, delicious, and it would keep the doctor away until the end of your long life.

But unfortunately, this just isn't the case. After years of clinical trials, the results are as confusing as they've ever been. No one can say for certain that taking replacement hormones on a long-term basis is safe, yet no one can claim that it's dangerous for every woman, either. Some studies indict estrogen as increasing cancer risk; some say it's the progestin that's the culprit. And other studies say that ERT or HRT has little effect on whether or not you'll develop cancer—because there are so many other variables to take into account. One additional wrinkle in the controversy is that women in America are so much more prone to developing heart disease than breast cancer, and estrogen does give a woman the edge on cardiovascular health. Unfortunately, adding the progestin in an HRT regimen may lower the cardiac benefits.

When making a judgment, the question has to be a

personal one. Is your risk of heart disease or osteoporosis great enough to warrant taking a medication that may increase your risk of breast and endometrial cancers, or gallbladder, liver, or kidney disease? But if you choose not to medicate, are you dooming yourself to an early or difficult death?

Some answers have come from the PEPI trial, a three-year study of nearly 900 women on various forms of hormone therapy, released in 1994. A great deal more information will come from a study by the Women's Health Initiative, a branch of the National Institutes of Health. Over a ten-year period, 140,000 women will be randomly assigned to different hormone therapies, and these will be compared with other factors such as diet and exercise in the prevention of degenerative diseases. Unfortunately, we have to wait until the year 2006 for these results to be published, at which point many of us will already be dealing with the problems inherent in taking or not taking this medication.

Will we ever know for sure if HRT is the correct choice for us—and how much we should take for how long? Right now, it's hard to say that there will ever be a definitive answer. Unless you had a crystal ball and could foresee the way that your body would change over time, it would be virtually impossible to gauge what you should do.

All of life involves risk. This chapter will attempt to make sense of the various statistics and predictions and relate them directly to you so that you can make a choice—even if it's only a temporary one—pro or con.

The Dispute Over Replacement Hormones

Experts are still tossing the ball back and forth—yes, you should; no, you shouldn't. No wonder it's so difficult for each of us to reach a personal decision that is comfortable. Let's examine the various sides of the argument.

Q: Why do some experts say I should be taking HRT?

Since every woman loses estrogen after menopause, her risks of developing and dying of heart disease and osteoporosis rise abruptly within a five- to seven-year period (or overnight, if she has had a surgical menopause). In order to gain maximum protection, she should be taking HRT, which will also alleviate the common and uncommon complaints of menopause.

The Brigham and Women's Hospital ten-year survey of 49,000 nurses showed that the probability of a white woman fifty to ninety-four years old dying of heart disease is 31 percent, as opposed to only 2.8 percent for breast cancer and hip fracture and 0.7 percent for endometrial cancer. Taking replacement hormones reduces her risk of heart disease to 25 percent and of hip fracture to 2.2 percent.

What about breast cancer? The lifetime probability of developing it is 1 in 8 women. The risk of getting breast cancer increases over time, so that the risk to a younger woman is lower than it is for an older woman. If women take HRT, they raise their risk by only 0.5 percent. The baseline on endometrial cancer is that 1 in 1,000 women will develop it, and taking HRT increases this risk by only 0.1 percent.

Q: Why do some experts say I shouldn't be taking HRT?

The body was not designed to keep manufacturing hormones at the same rate throughout its lifetime. There were many women of previous generations who lived to ripe old ages and never succumbed to heart disease or osteoporosis. The antimedication theorists feel that it's not natural to alter the endocrine status of a fifty- or sixty-year-old body. They also argue that even the slightest possibility of an elevated risk of breast and other cancers is enough to rule out HRT.

Another point they make is that you may be risking cancer for what amounts to a very small increase in life expectancy. Treatment with HRT extends the life of a woman with heart disease or osteoporosis by only a few months.

Q: Why can't anyone agree?

Studies are done by different research scientists who use different populations and different dosages of different medications to prove similar theories. Some studies lump together all women who've ever taken estrogen, even though part of this group may only have stayed on the medication for nine months or a year. Many of the results are not statistically significant—that is, there isn't a huge gap between health or disease of users or nonusers. Also, it's harder for negative results to get published, which means that when a metanalysis (a grouping of several studies) is done, it's usually heavily weighted on the HRT-is-good-for-you side. Research physicians usually don't have a clinical practice and are unaware of the experiences of most ordinary women who decide to take this medication on their own.

How Many Risks? How Many Benefits?

There is no cut-and-dried measurement scale, because each woman's situation is different. But you can start to make an evaluation on whether or not HRT is right for you based on the following information.

Q: All theories aside, what risks have been reported on this therapy?

Studies have shown that women who take HRT can increase their risk of endometrial cancer and may also increase their risk of breast cancer (although the breast cancer issue is highly controversial, and many other variables are involved). Some studies show that women on HRT may be at higher risk for stroke and may also have a higher tendency to develop elevated blood pressure, benign liver tumors, gallstones, and kidney disease.

Q: What are the major benefits of this therapy?

ERT and HRT have been shown to save lives. In a study done in 1988 that added up deaths due to ischemic heart disease and osteoporotic hip fractures, it was shown that there would be fewer deaths per year if more women took hormones after menopause. In women sixty-five to seventy-four who used HRT, less than 211 per 100,000 would die of these causes and in those who used ERT it was less than 328 per 100,000.

Women who got breast cancer after having been on HRT appeared to fare much better in treatment and to have better survival rates than those who developed breast cancer and were not on HRT.

Another plus is that quality of life improves for many women who take this medication. They experience fewer hot flashes, joint pains, and other unpleasant symptoms; they enjoy a more comfortable sex life; and they feel less fatigue on a day-to-day basis.

Q: What are common side effects of taking HRT, and are any of them life-threatening?

Side effects include weight gain, stomach upset, elevation in blood pressure, increase in size of fibroids, migraine headaches, PMS symptoms (bloating, water retention, tender breasts), breakthrough bleeding (bleeding unrelated to a regular period), allergic reactions, varicose veins, thinning hair or hair loss, anxiety, and other symptoms that may be difficult to describe but which make a woman feel out of control of her body.

The only one of these that could be life-threatening is the elevation in blood pressure. It is possible that an adjustment in brand of drug, dosage, or administration will take care of some or all of these side effects.

Q: All the information I get from my doctor talks about "relative risks." What does that mean?

A relative risk deals with the probability involved with just one variable—let's take the example of the risk of breast cancer occurring in a group of people who are in a study. A relative risk is the incidence of disease among those who have been exposed to one risk factor (which might be either smoking, eating fatty foods, or taking HRT), divided by the incidence of disease among those who haven't been exposed. Relative risk changes over time.

An absolute risk, on the other hand, weighs all factors together—if your father died at forty of a heart attack, if you are a sixty-three-year-old overweight woman, if you don't exercise and smoke two packs a day, your absolute risk of developing heart disease is exceptionally high. You can change some of the factors (which will influence the risk slightly), but others remain unchanged.

Q: What are the risks I run by taking HRT on a short-term basis?

There has been no indication that you run any risk at all by taking estrogen alone or estrogen plus a progestin for less than five years. If your intention is simply to alleviate menopausal complaints for the few years that they bother you, you will not be doing yourself any future harm and will undoubtedly feel that the quality of your life has improved.

Q: How do my risks increase after taking HRT over five years?

After five years on the medication, risk of developing breast cancer rises on average 30 to 70 percent (this percentage may be higher depending on the population studied and the type or dose they were on). The risk is increasingly higher if you have been on the drug for ten to fifteen years. This risk—three and a half times that of nonusers—remains high even six years after you've discontinued hormone use.

Q: Are there any circumstances that would make it dangerous for me to take HRT?

A known or suspected estrogen-dependent breast or uterine cancer, or having one or more primary relatives (your mother or sisters) who had breast cancer before they reached menopause would be the most compelling reason not to take replacement hormones. Abnormal or unexplained genital bleeding would prohibit use, as would chronic liver or kidney disease. It is also questionable whether you should take hormones if you have any type of blood clotting problems or have had a stroke (although some physicians would prescribe a patch rather than an oral regimen to someone with this type of medical history).

Estrogen Alone or Estrogen Plus a Progestin— What's Safer?

The statistics show that the most successful uses of hormone therapy are for women who have no uterus—and therefore don't have to worry about endometrial cancer. Their drug regimen, estrogen only, gives the highest benefits with the least risk. But what about a woman with an intact uterus who must take a progestin to protect her endometrium?

Q: Why is ERT safer than HRT?
If you have no uterus (and therefore no endometrium), you have eliminated your risk of endometrial cancer. You need only take estrogen to protect your heart and bones and alleviate menopausal complaints. By eliminating the need for a progestin, you get better lipid profiles (ERT raises HDL and lowers LDL; HRT only raises HDL). Also, you eliminate the concern raised by the studies that relate the progestin (which can increase breast cell proliferation) to high breast cancer risk.

The progestin component of hormone replacement therapy is also the one that most women find uncomfortable—it frequently causes PMS symptoms such as bloating, breast tenderness, water retention, and depression.

Q: So does that mean that estrogen by itself is completely safe?
No one can say that for sure. Various cancers grow under the influence of estrogen, so the more of it there is in the body, the higher the risk of certain cells changing in an abnormal fashion. Women who have already had estrogen-dependent cancers are not generally good candidates for ERT or HRT.

Q: If I only take ERT, does the dosage of estrogen make a difference?
Yes. A daily dose of 0.625 mg estrogen for under five years does not increase the risk of breast cancer. However, a daily dose of 1.25 mg may increase the risk of breast

cancer, particularly if you're taking a higher dosage for more than five years.

Q: If I'm concerned about the risks of taking a progestin, can I take just estrogen?

Not if you still have an intact uterus. Although some physicians will allow you to skip one or even two months of the progestin, a proliferation in endometrial tissue has been charted after only seventy-two days on unopposed estrogen.

Q: If I have to take a progestin, will this increase my risk of heart disease?

Rather than raising your risk, having the progestin seems to diminish the benefits you might have had on an estrogen-only regimen. (This is not the case with natural progesterone, which keeps HDLs high.)

Q: Will taking the progestin make a difference if I'm at risk for osteoporosis?

There have been no definitive studies yet to show that the progestin or natural progesterone makes a big difference in bone resorption.

Q: What is the difference in risk between taking natural micronized progesterone and a synthetic progestin?

The PEPI trials indicate that natural micronized progesterone plus estrogen give better lipid profiles than synthetic progestin plus estrogen. It is not yet known whether this effect translates into lower disease risks. No trials have yet shown that natural progesterone is less likely to increase breast cancer risk than the synthetic. And the real problem here is that, since much of the product is custom-compounded in private pharmacies, there is no guarantee of consistency or potency. If you have a uterus, you should certainly be concerned about getting enough benefit to keep the lining of the uterus from proliferating. If your dosage of natural progesterone is too low, you may be more at risk for endometrial cancer than if you took the synthetic progestin.

Specific Risk Factors to Consider

The risk for one individual isn't always pertinent to another, but it's important to know what the national averages are for risks of breast, endometrial, and ovarian cancer, and for liver, gallbladder, and kidney disease when you are making your decision about whether or not to take HRT.

Q: What is my risk of developing breast cancer?
One in eight women in the United States will develop breast cancer during her lifetime. Breast cancer risk increases with age, and this is true both of women who are taking hormones and those who are not. The risk also increases if you are obese, if you have always eaten a high-fat diet, or if you had an early puberty, a late menopause, or never had children.

The breast responds differently to hormonal stimulation after menopause. The older breast seems more sensitive to both the estrogen produced by the body and to that added in a medication.

Estrogen interacts with various tissues (such as the breast, the uterus, the skin, the bone, and the heart) and gives them the go-ahead to produce more cells. When these cells proliferate, there is always the possibility that some could mutate and start growing abnormally. This doesn't happen in every case or, indeed, in most cases. But in some cases, too much estrogen in the breast can mean cancer.

Studies that compare breast cancer risk in hysterectomized women on ERT and women with an intact uterus on HRT don't always draw neat conclusions on whether the estrogen or progestin is the culprit. On the one hand, too much estrogen in the breast creates a lot of cell activity; on the other, progestin may be implicated in breast changes as well, because these changes—whether they are normal or abnormal—occur during the luteal phase of the rep·oductive cycle, when progesterone is the predominant hormone.

A 1992 study from the University of California, San Francisco, and the San Francisco Kaiser Permanente Medical Center analyzed the risks of various different cancers. Their results are those quoted throughout this chapter.

A fifty-year-old white woman has a 10 percent lifetime probability of developing breast cancer and a 3 percent probability of dying of this disease. The median age of developing breast cancer is sixty-nine years. If this woman, however, has a family history of breast cancer, her lifetime probability jumps to 19.3 percent of developing it and her median life expectancy is shortened by six months.

Taking estrogen is estimated to increase the lifetime probability of developing breast cancer to 24.1 percent and this risk increases slightly if the dosage is higher than 0.625 mg daily for a period of longer than five years.

The risk of developing breast cancer if you take estrogen plus progestin is slightly higher the longer you take it. Data are very inconsistent, however, on how much influence the progestin has.

Q: What is my risk of developing endometrial cancer?

A fifty-year-old white woman has a 2.6 percent lifetime risk of developing endometrial cancer. But because this problem is easily detectable and treatable, her risk of dying of this cancer is only 3 in 1,000. The median age at which endometrial cancer develops is sixty-eight years.

The risk of developing this cancer is greatly reduced, and in most cases eliminated, if a progestin is taken along with estrogen.

Q: What is my risk of developing gallbladder, liver, or kidney disease?

Gallstones are made of cholesterol and other fatty substances in bile, and they typically affect overweight, light-haired women before or during the climacteric. Taking estrogen doubles your chances of developing gallstones, but usually only if you take the oral medication. The reason is that the hormone must be metabolized by the liver, and therefore affects the liver's excretory function. The estrogen patch was designed to eliminate "first-pass" problems with the liver.

How would you suspect that you might have gallstones? Be aware of frequent indigestion and nausea, accompanied by pain in the upper part of your abdomen.

The kidney, along with the liver, is also responsible for processing and removing toxins and other chemicals from the body. If these organs have to work too hard, as they do when metabolizing or excreting additional estrogen and progesterone, they can begin to show signs of damage.

Risks of Not Taking HRT

On the other hand, if you don't take this medication, what diseases and conditions might you develop along the way? What ultimate difference will they make in your quality and quantity of life? Let's examine the possibilities.

Q: What is my risk of developing heart disease?

Women who aren't at high risk for coronary artery disease have a 31 percent risk of dying of a heart attack, and taking HRT apparently reduces that risk by 20 percent. It cuts in half the probability of developing coronary disease—although adding a progestin to estrogen therapy gives a somewhat lower reduction in risk.

A fifty-year-old high-risk woman (who has diagnosed heart disease or has had a heart attack) has an 83.9 percent lifetime probability of recurrent heart disease and a life expectancy that is about seven years less than a woman who isn't at high risk. Taking HRT would reduce her lifetime risk to 76.4 percent.

Q: What is my risk of developing osteoporosis and dying of complications of a hip fracture?

A fifty-year-old white woman has a 15 percent lifetime possibility of fracturing a hip, and a 1.5 percent probability of dying of complications of that fracture. Her median age of first hip fracture is seventy-nine.

But if she is at high risk for osteoporosis because of low bone mineral density, her estimated lifetime probability of hip fracture jumps to 36.2 percent, and her median life expectancy is shorter by five months as compared to women with normal bone density.

Treatment with estrogen would reduce the probability of hip fracture to 31.4 percent and extend life expectancy by one year.

Q: What is my risk of dying of a stroke?

A fifty-year-old woman has a 20 percent lifetime probability of developing and an 8 percent probability of dying of stroke. The median age of death from stroke is eighty-three years.

It's not at all certain how taking HRT changes the picture. However, many women with blood clotting problems are advised not to take hormone replacement, certainly not the oral medication. Since certain strokes occur because of clots that form and travel to the brain, HRT may be inadvisable for those women at high risk for stroke.

However, it must also be noted that some data show *fewer* deaths from stroke among HRT users. The final word on HRT and stroke is still to be decided.

Personal Lives: Personal Decisions

Every woman is different. Their stories make up the vast literature—which is still growing—of case histories that relate to hormone replacement therapy.

Q: I've been on cyclic HRT for three years and just started having breakthrough bleeding in addition to my regular monthly withdrawal "period." How should I make the decision whether or not to stay on the medication?

Your doctor will advise performing a transvaginal ultrasound to check the thickness of your endometrium and may wish to do an endometrial biopsy to rule out endometrial cancer. S/he'll also do a hemoglobin count to see if you're anemic. If you have no abnormalities, an adjustment in dosage or brand of product may stop the bleeding.

Q: I had my ovaries removed when I was thirty-six because of a cyst that apparently was borderline cancerous. I've been taking ERT ever since. Now, at fifty-two, I wonder if I've "caught up" to most of my friends whose ovaries have lost their ability to produce estrogen. Can I stop taking the medication and use alternative treatments for improved health like diet, exercise, and herbs?

You should consult your physician and explain that you would prefer to use natural therapies if possible. You should discuss having a bone densitometry test and an EKG to make sure that your heart and bones are healthy. If your doctor gives you the okay, you should wean yourself off ERT slowly and begin your alternative treatments at the same time, so as not to bring on hot flashes, vaginal dryness, and other common menopausal complaints.

Q: I'm very overweight (285 pounds on a five-foot six-inch body), and I know this is bad for my health. But my sister had breast cancer, and I wonder, Should I take HRT?

Because of your weight, you have a high number of fat cells, which convert your adrenal hormones into estrone, a weaker form of estrogen. You are at higher risk for heart disease because you are heavy, but you also have higher estrogen levels, which protect your heart. Since you are also at higher risk for breast cancer, this is the marker to consider. The best course of action is to get on a strict diet and exercise program and rule out HRT for now. You may wish to reconsider it when you're down to a healthy weight.

Q: I had endometrial cancer and had a hysterectomy seven years ago. I have been consistently cancer-free in exams since then. My mother died of complications of a hip fracture, and though I've really been trying to stop, I'm still an infrequent smoker. Would it be wise for me to start ERT?

Your oncologist would probably say no, but your gynecologist and endocrinologist would say that, under certain circumstances, and depending on the particular type of cancer you had, you're going to be okay on this therapy.

They might go so far as to say that it's a good idea for you to take ERT, because you still need to protect your heart and bones as you age. You should, of course, get into a smoking-cessation program and stick with it.

Q: I had a lumpectomy and radiation therapy for breast cancer three years ago. Should I ever consider taking HRT?

This would completely depend on the characteristics of your cancer. If the cancer was estrogen-dependent and/or had spread to your lymph nodes, you should not be on HRT. However, if your cancer was not estrogen-dependent and you wait another two years to be certain the cancer doesn't reappear, you might consider HRT. Some physicians would give you the nod; others would say that you should avoid it. Treating a previous cancer patient with HRT is still very controversial.

Q: I've always had fibrocystic breasts, but when the lumps were aspirated, I found out that they were benign. Should I consider HRT?

Most doctors are in agreement that the type of cells that develop into cysts generally do not develop into cancers. Therefore, they would approve HRT for a woman with fibrocystic breast disease unless aspiration or lumpectomy proved that cancerous cells were present.

Q: I had a hysterectomy five years ago at forty-five because of an enlarged fibroid that was pressing on my bladder—but I still have my ovaries. I am not at risk for either heart disease or osteoporosis. I never smoked, I eat a very low-fat diet, and I exercise daily. I'm not troubled by hot flashes or vaginal dryness. Should I be on ERT?

You are at slightly higher-than-normal risk for heart disease without a uterus, because blood flow to the ovaries—which supply estrogen—is severed during this surgery, making you slightly estrogen-deficient. However, you're a very healthy individual, and the only glitch in your background was fibroids, which grow under the influence of estrogen. Your physician may suggest ERT now, but s/he may also counsel you to wait. Continue your excellent self-care and have a densitometry test and a retest of your cholesterol levels in a couple of years to see how your bones and lipid levels are doing. If you're still in the normal range, you may want to wait ten years before you think about HRT.

Q: I feel too nervous to put hormones into my body for three or four decades. Could I wait ten years and start HRT when I'm more at risk for disease and need protection?

The thinking used to be that, for prevention of osteoporosis and probably for heart disease, the best course of action was to start HRT within three years of menopause and continue until death. Discontinuing this medication—no matter how long you've been on it—means losing all the benefit you've gained to your bone mass and to your lipid profile.

But these days, because it's clear that the longer you're on HRT the greater your cancer risk, many physicians think it may be prudent to wait several years and see. Maybe at fifty your densitometry readings are just under normal, but by sixty, you are at -2.5 and really need some intervention to reduce fracture risk. Short-term studies show that increases in bone density after taking HRT are small at menopause but may be substantial in older women with greater losses in bone mass and density. So, some physicians feel that ten years after menopause might be a good time to begin treatment. Meanwhile, you would have saved yourself ten years of exposure to additional estrogen and breast cancer risk.

The same holds true when you're thinking about HRT for your heart. Although coronary artery disease is the number one killer of women in this country, most of these women are elderly, not menopausal. In 1994, 86,000 women between fifty-five and seventy-four died of heart disease, but 260,000 women over seventy-five died of heart disease. This means that if you stick with your excellent diet, exercise, and stress-reduction programs, and then start HRT ten years from now, you may reap the combined benefits of nonmedical and medical therapies.

Weighing Risks and Benefits

The bottom line is still fuzzy. There are so many possibilities, and although you know you have to prioritize your health needs, it's hard to really know what should come first in your decision-making process. Let's analyze the data—but let's also keep your personal factors at the top of your list.

Q: How do I find out what my risks are?
Get a complete medical checkup and have your doctor obtain a report on your HDL and LDL cholesterol levels, your triglyceride levels and total cholesterol, and serum glucose levels. Get an EKG to be certain that your heart is in good shape, and if your physician feels it's warranted, get a bone densitometry test and see where you stand in comparison to women your age. If you are past fifty, you should also have a mammogram.

Q: How do I weigh the various risks I might have of dying of various diseases?
First, remember that your risk factors and lifestyle factors cannot possibly match any particular group that's been measured. You may have a strong family history of disease, yet eat less fat and exercise more than members of a trial study; you may have smoked or been anorectic at

one point in your life but corrected those problems; you may be an avid practitioner of meditation or yoga that might change the probability of your dying of a certain disease at a certain age.

But if you're going by national standards (and that's the best "ruler" we've got), a pretty common standard measurement of how you are likely to die shows that you have a much greater risk of dying of a heart attack than anything else. For postmenopausal women, the lifetime risk of dying of a heart attack is 31 percent; that of dying of breast cancer is 2.8 percent; and that of dying of endometrial cancer is less than 1 percent.

A recent study of five hundred women at the Kaiser Permanente Medical Care Program in Oakland, California, who had taken HRT for more than twenty years was very positive about the advantages of this therapy. By taking HRT, a woman reduces her risk of dying *from any cause* by 46 percent. She reduces her risk of dying of a heart attack by 60 percent.

Although there was a slightly higher rate of breast cancer in estrogen users, it was statistically offset by the lower death rate from lung cancer.

Q: I'm still so confused. How do I weigh all the risks against the benefits?

The only way to make your choice is to weigh your personal factors and ask yourself serious questions about your life, your health (good and bad), and your fears and hopes for the future.

Our image of a heart attack is that of a final, crushing blow; cancer, on the other hand, seems like a lingering evil. In fact, most women don't have heart attacks as their first symptom but rather struggle for years with a debilitating, painful heart condition. Cancer, on the other hand, if treated promptly and aggressively, can go into remission and in many cases never reappear. So neither illness can be painted as better or worse.

If you have no family history of either heart disease or cancer, and you're just going by the national standard, you are more likely to die of a heart attack than cancer. But if you take a medication that increases a risk, those statistics change. The National Institutes of Health Cancer Review in 1992 reported that an average woman who dies of heart disease loses eight years on her projected life expectancy. An average woman who dies of breast cancer, however, loses nineteen years of her projected life expectancy. This means that if you opt not to take HRT and protect your heart, you still may live a longer life than if you medicated yourself for several decades and developed cancer as a result.

Q: Are there any assurances that the decision I make today will keep me safe?

None at all—because your risks change over time. And perhaps that's the real answer to the big question of whether or not it's safe to take HRT. *It is safe for some women at certain times of their lives.*

Here are your choices:

Do nothing now. If you are in good health and have few or no risk factors and your EKG and bone densitometry tests indicated that you are in the normal range, sit tight and start a vigorous program of good nutrition, supplementation, exercise, and stress management. Reconsider your decision if your risk factors change.

Start HRT now for a limited time. If you are seriously bothered by menopausal complaints, take low-dose HRT, possibly using one of the more "natural" products that derives its estrogen from estrone sulfate rather than estradiol, for five years or less. (See Chapter 7 for your options.)

Start HRT now and continue indefinitely. If you have multiple risk factors and feel you should protect your heart and bones when you can, then take hormones. You can still decide to stop at any point, although it does mean that you will lose the benefit that you have gained.

Start HRT at sixty-five when your risks are high. If you remain in good health for the next fifteen or twenty years, you can at that point make the choice to start hormones to protect your heart and bones.

Chapter Six

Finding the Right Physician and Other Health Care Providers

If you are still seeing the same family doctor you had when you were a teenager or the same ob/gyn who delivered your children, you may want to think seriously about getting some fresh opinions about your health care. It often pays to consult the physician who most frequently sees people like you. This individual is going to be more interested in the concerns of midlife women, will have more recent and up-to-date knowledge of their health care, and may offer innovative procedures and programs that you can take advantage of. There's also something reassuring about sitting quietly in a waiting room *without* hordes of little kids running around, yelling, and playing.

You need a person you can really talk to, someone who will be receptive to answering the questions in this book and others that will come to mind as you think more seriously about what course of action you wish to take with your menopause and your decision about HRT. You need to see a professional who is comfortable discussing difficult issues such as sexuality and aging; you need to have guidelines so that you can maintain your regular gynecological health and general health—mental as well as physical; you need to know which tests might be appropriate for you at this time of life, to ascertain your possible risks for osteoporosis and heart disease.

The Right Physician for You in Midlife

Most people will interview at least three different contractors to get a quote for home renovation, but how many of us really make a determined and knowledgeable search for a good doctor? When selecting a physician to guide you through menopause and beyond, when looking for someone who can help you make the best choice about HRT, ERT, and/or complementary treatments, you need to be thorough and exacting.

Q: Is it okay to stay with the ob/gyn I've had since my first child was born?

Perhaps—it all depends on who your doctor is. If your ob/gyn is still mostly involved with reproductive-aged women and his or her office is decorated top to toe with baby pictures, this could mean that you need someone more attuned to your needs. Midlife gynecologists and endocrinologists are not only up to the moment on the latest information about HRT, osteoporosis, heart disease, and aging, but they may also have an office and diagnostic equipment designed for your current health requirements.

You might also think about switching if you sense that your physician just isn't interested in the concerns of midlife women. The attitude of your professional can do a lot to foster a better health care relationship with patients and to encourage you to get as much good information as you can about how to help yourself.

Q: If I decide to switch, how do I figure out what type of doctor I should see?

You should always interview several new doctors and consider whether the person you're looking for will be your primary care physician or a specialist. You will want to see a family doctor with a strong interest in midlife women if you want primary care and a gynecologist or endocrinologist for specialized care. If you're about to undergo a difficult surgical procedure such as a hysterectomy, mastectomy, or coronary bypass, you should have a second opinion by a gynecological surgeon, a breast surgeon, or a cardiologist and cardiac surgeon. (Most insurance companies require one anyway.)

Q: Does it make a difference whether I see a male or a female physician?

This is a very personal choice. However, gender doesn't necessarily make a difference—it's the particular woman or man you're seeing that's important.

A report in the *New England Journal of Medicine* indicated that women who see women doctors tend to have more mammograms and Pap smears than those who see male doctors—possibly because a woman who needs a procedure herself will be more likely to prescribe it for others. Women doctors also tend to suggest starting HRT more than men—and this can be a mixed blessing. Because they are concerned about their patients' long-term well-being, they want to offer them the option of this therapy; however, some may be so enthusiastic they recommend it for all patients rather than on a case-by-case basis.

Some women who have been sexually traumatized in earlier life feel more comfortable with a female physician. And some who have had difficult relationships with male doctors in the past may also select a female for midlife care.

However, it should be pointed out that many male doctors who are currently going into practice are extremely sensitive to women's issues. An innovative and compassionate person of either gender is a good choice for the midlife woman.

Q: Does it matter whether my doctor is young or old?
Probably not. There are physicians who finished their training thirty years ago who are just as or more up-to-date on midlife issues than those right out of their residency. It is true, however, that some physicians of both sexes with growing families of their own have decided to opt out of reproductive medicine because they don't want to have to get up in the middle of the night and deliver babies if they have their own babies at home to attend to. This means they may have more inclination to care for the older woman and, consequently, more expertise in midlife care because of extensive training in that area.

Q: What credentials should a midlife women's doctor have?
Your doctor should have completed his or her training in an institution accredited by the ACGME (Accreditation Council for Graduate Medical Education) in a program accredited by one of several RRCs (Residency Review Committees for either Internal Medicine, Ob/Gyn, or Family Practice). Institutions offering such training (usually universities or large hospitals) are strictly regulated. He or she must be licensed by the state.

Most of the doctors you'll be interested in consulting will have completed significant training after medical school: a year of internship, two to five years of residency or training in their specialty, and possibly one to three years of a fellowship, which is further specialty training involving laboratory work. After completing this course and working in the field for a year or two, the individual will have to pass written and oral examinations and become board certified. (A doctor doesn't have to be board certified to practice, but this credential certainly indicates the good preparation a doctor has had.)

Which specialties should you consider? Most women in midlife selecting a physician will want a gynecologist, an obstetrician/gynecologist, or an endocrinologist. If you are interested in holistic health, you may wish to consult an osteopath or a naturopath who has experience with midlife women.

Q: How do I find a doctor who will listen as well as talk to me?

Schedule consultations with a few physicians before you make a final choice. A doctor should be interested in what you have to say and who you are as a person—not just in the symptoms you present with. Being a whiz at a physical exam is great, but if s/he can't conduct a two-way conversation when you're sitting up clothed in the consultation room, this is not the physician for you.

Making the Most of Your Doctor's Appointments

It's not enough just to show up at your appointments—you have to be an active participant in your own health care. The more you know what you want from your physician, the better care you'll get.

Q: What should I do to prepare for my first appointment with a new doctor?

Do your homework. Make sure you know your medical history (or if you're switching doctors, have your former physician fax all your records to the new one prior to your first appointment).

Make a list of all the medications you take. Include vitamins, nutritional supplements, herbs, homeopathic remedies, and all over-the-counter medications as well.

Take a notebook with you. You can write down all the questions you have for the doctor in advance and take notes during your consultation on the information s/he gives you. It's easy to get anxious in a doctor's examining room and not remember crucial information about symptoms, lifestyle changes, and treatments, or dosages, side effects, and contraindications of medications s/he might have prescribed.

Find out particulars about test results and follow-up exams. Be sure to ask if there is a particular time of day when it's good to call in with additional questions. (Some physicians have early-morning hotline numbers you can call.)

Q: What are some signs that I am getting adequate care?

A few hints will point the way:

- The office interview should be private, with no telephone interruptions or assistants running in with requests.
- The doctor should have a routine list of medical and personal questions to ask and then should turn the floor over to you so that you can ask questions about the way s/he handles patients, wellness, and illness. He or she should answer you without defensiveness.
- The physical exam should feel comfortable to you. Pay attention to the way the doctor explains diagnostic procedures, treatments, and medications. Does s/he warm the speculum before inserting it? Does

s/he tell you which organs s/he is going to be touching before touching them? Is a nurse or physician's assistant present at the exam? (Some short-staffed offices will only provide this service if you request it—but they must provide it!)

- The doctor should take your concerns into consideration. Does s/he really listen and allow you time to air all the issues you consider important?

- If a referral to a specialist is needed, your doctor should check back with you to find out how you liked the other physician and how you think the office visit went. Does s/he make the effort to continue to consult with the specialist to be certain that the care you need is being provided?

- You should feel good about being with this doctor and feel comfortable with the kind of attention you're getting. Sometimes, intuition will lead you to the choice of a person who is uniquely qualified to care for you.

Asking Your Physician About HRT or ERT

One of the big decisions you have to make—whether you make it now or several years from now—is whether you will take medication to replace the hormones you are losing as you pass through menopause. An informed physician who understands you and your health care goals can be a great asset at this time of life.

Q: Will my doctor tell me I have to take HRT whether I need it or not?

The medical establishment really has no consensus about whether every woman past menopause should be taking replacement hormones, but the great majority of general practitioners, family physicians, gynecologists, and cardiologists are for it. The great majority of oncologists and naturopathic and holistic medicine physicians are against it. Of course, there are exceptions in every category.

There is no reason for your doctor to be eager for you to be on this therapy prior to checking out your general health, your motivations for taking HRT, and your health concerns other than medication. It is no longer a given that *all* women past menopause should necessarily take HRT—so it's important to know that your doctor wants to find out (just as you do) if it's the right choice for you.

Most doctors—whatever their background—do say that HRT is not for everyone, and that each woman's situation and needs are unique and must be carefully evaluated.

If you come into your doctor's office complaining that you feel lousy, you can't sleep because of night sweats, you've lost interest in sex, your clothes are drenched every hour on the hour, and you need help—QUICK—he or she will probably strongly suggest trying hormones for a few months to see if the therapy makes a difference. This is not an ideal way to make your HRT decision.

Instead, you should come in armed with information, arguments pro and con, and debate the issues with your doctor. You may have some gut feelings about the matter, but come with an open mind. Be willing to accept new ideas and theories. It's important to air your feelings, but you need a factual basis for your decision, which can be determined by the results of diagnostic tests. Your doctor can find out the exact status of your heart and bones through these tests. Only then can you set your priorities for your healthy future.

If you are interested in trying a holistic approach before you consider medication to see if it makes a difference in your general health, you must also broach this subject with your doctor. It's conceivable that s/he won't suggest a revamped diet and exercise program, tai chi and meditation, as well as an herbal or vitamin-mineral supplement simply because he or she is not familiar with this type of preventive medicine and hasn't seen the results in patients. It will be up to you to find alternative therapists who can work in cooperation with your primary care physician.

If you do try the natural therapies, and they haven't made you more comfortable after three months, or if you are deeply concerned about your risk factors for heart disease or osteoporosis, then the decision for starting HRT is your next logical choice.

Q: How will my doctor and I know if HRT is right for me?

If you are at high risk for heart disease or osteoporosis or have a strong family history of either, you should probably be on medication.

If you have already suffered a heart attack, you are a very good candidate for HRT, since you can drastically improve your cholesterol levels with this medication and possibly prevent a second attack.

If you are debilitated by symptoms (hot flashes that keep you up all night, vaginal dryness that has wrecked your sex life, joint pains, depression, or fatigue) that make it difficult for you to live an active life, your physician will probably suggest HRT.

If you have had a hysterectomy and any of the above conditions or symptoms pertain to you, your physician will also probably feel that a course of HRT is warranted. You have a safer prognosis on the medication than a woman with a uterus since you only need estrogen and not estrogen plus a progestin (which could lower the protective value of estrogen on your cardiovascular system).

Q: What kinds of preparation and testing would my doctor order before I start HRT?

Your doctor will want to check you out thoroughly before prescribing medication.

He or she will take a thorough family history if you haven't done one yet, with special emphasis on personal and family information about osteoporosis, heart disease, and cancer. You'd then have a full physical, including a pelvic exam with a Pap smear and a breast exam. You would also have a mammogram at this time if you haven't had one for two years, or one year if you're over fifty. Your doctor may suggest a bone densitometry test and an EKG, depending on your history.

Your doctor will also wish to do a complete battery of blood tests for blood sugar (glucose) levels, thyroid function, liver function, cholesterol and triglyceride levels, and calcium and phosphorus levels.

When all the results are back, this is the time to sit down and seriously discuss why HRT is a good option for you now, or whether you should wait several months or a year and then consider medication.

Q: Does timing make a difference? How do I know if I should start HRT now, or next year, or ten years from now?

If you've been having irregular periods or have stopped menstruating, if you are troubled by hot flashes and vaginal dryness, your physician may suggest a blood test to determine the ratio of FSH (follicle-stimulating hormone) to estradiol (endogenous estrogen) in your system. If the FSH is greater than 40 and your estradiol is less than 14, you might benefit from HRT, particularly if your symptoms have been disrupting your lifestyle or you're at high risk for osteoporosis or heart disease.

Some physicians will do a vaginal ultrasound or endometrial biopsy before starting you on medication, to check the condition of your endometrium and make sure that it has no abnormal cells that might proliferate under the influence of estrogen.

Some physicians will give a "progesterone challenge test," where you take 10 mg progesterone for seven to ten days. When you discontinue the hormone, you should bleed if you have adequate levels of estrogen in your body. If you don't bleed, that's an indication that you could use replacement estrogen and might be ready to start HRT.

Some physicians will do no tests at all, particularly if you've been on a low-dose birth control pill and are in your mid- to late forties. They will simply switch you over to the lowest dosage of HRT and see how you do for three months. At the end of that time, you should check in with your doctor to reevaluate your dosage and regimen.

Q: How often should I follow up with my doctor on my HRT medication schedule?

Most gynecologists would like to see you every six months for eighteen months or two years, after which you'll taper off to visits once a year. At these appointments, you can discuss your medication, dosage, and changes in your health status. If you are having any trouble with side effects, or the medication is not alleviating your symptoms, you should certainly check in sooner than that. Especially when you first start this medication, you should be in close touch to ascertain the lowest dosage that will do the job.

Q: What do I do if I want to discontinue HRT?

Talk to your doctor. If you are troubled by side effects, or if you feel the medication isn't having an effect on your symptoms, the first step is to reevaluate the amount or particular type of medication you're taking. It's possible that by lowering or raising the dosage or switching products, you can alleviate the problems you're having.

But if that doesn't work, and you're feeling bloated and uncomfortable, or you are concerned about staying on HRT because you've gained weight or your blood pressure is elevated, you and your physician will want to discuss how to wean you off the drugs slowly. (See Chapter 7 for a discussion of how to taper off HRT.)

Q: What do I do if I disagree with my doctor about my medication or treatment?

Because doctors have a lot more training than lay-people, we tend to assume that they know best, especially when it comes to what drugs we take. This is partly, but not entirely, true. You know yourself, and your physical and emotional reactions should guide you when you're making an assessment of your health care. If something feels wrong, it probably *is* wrong.

However, if your doctor insists his or her way is *the* way and refuses to consider your concerns, you are entitled to get a second opinion.

The Midlife Exam—Tests and Recommendations

HRT is only one of your concerns at this time of life. If you are strong in body and mind, you are in a better position to deal with life—on estrogen or off it. If you haven't had a full checkup since your last child was born, this is the time to get one. You may also need some specialized diagnostic procedures to help your physician ascertain your current health status.

Q: What should a regular gynecological exam at midlife consist of?

The exam should begin with a routine weight, blood

pressure, and heart rate check, as well as a urine sample to test for sugar and protein.

The physical should consist of an examination of your breasts and torso, and a palpation (touching and pressing) of your stomach and pelvic region. The next part of the exam should check your external organs (inner and outer labia and clitoris), and the bimanual exam should check your vagina, cervix, uterus, and ovaries. With one or two fingers inside you and one hand outside on the pelvic girdle, the doctor should manipulate the organs and ask whether you feel any discomfort.

Then, inserting a speculum, s/he should check those organs visually and do a Pap smear if you need one at that time. S/he should then withdraw the speculum and finish with a digital rectal exam to check for hemorrhoids, polyps, or anal fissures.

Q: How often should I have a Pap smear and mammogram?

A Pap smear should be done every year in a midlife woman to check for cervical cancer. A baseline mammogram should be performed at thirty-nine, then every two to three years until after your fiftieth birthday, after which time it should be done annually unless you have a family history of breast cancer—in which case it should be done annually from thirty-nine on. Although insurance carriers insist that mammograms are generally a waste of time and money in women under fifty, the American Cancer Society argues that any early cancer detection that results from vigilant checking is worth it.

Q: What's a transvaginal ultrasound test?

Sonograms use ultrasound waves to check the lining of the uterus to be certain that there is no overgrowth of cells. During this noninvasive procedure, a probe is inserted into the vagina and passed into the uterus. This probe scans the endometrium and checks its thickness by ultrasound waves.

Q: What's an endometrial biopsy?

During this office procedure, a small tube is inserted through the cervix into the uterus and suction is used to trap cells for later examination under a microscope. Some physicians dilate the cervix and use an instrument to take a sample—which can feel quite uncomfortable. Since this is an invasive procedure, you should ask your doctor whether the test is absolutely necessary and whether an ultrasound would suffice.

Q: If I'm concerned about osteoporosis, what tests would my physician order?

If you have lost significant height (an inch or two) in the last few years, or if you have a pronounced kyphosis (dowager's hump), if you have broken bones in the past during minor falls, if you have a strong family history of osteoporosis, or if you are experiencing medical problems that might put you at risk of osteoporosis, your doctor may wish to check the mass and density of your bones.

Blood tests would be done to measure red and white blood cell counts, as well as protein, calcium, thyroid and parathyroid hormone levels, and vitamin D levels. Gonadal hormone levels will tell your doctor how much estrogen you're still producing, and how that balances with the amount of follicle-stimulating hormone and luteinizing hormone your brain is making (see Chapter 2 for a full explanation of these hormones).

Your urine should also be tested. A twenty-four-hour urinary calcium and creatinine excretion test will determine whether you are losing calcium instead of absorbing it so that it can assist in the bone remodeling process.

The most important test for osteoporosis is the bone densitometry test. Some physicians routinely ask their patients to take this, whether or not they have any of the above symptoms, in order to help them make the choice for HRT.

The test uses a radiographic picture to measure the bone mineral content and density of the spine, hip, or forearm, and then compares the results to those of younger women (with "peak" bone mass) and samples of women your own age. Most women lose about 1 to 2 percent of their bone mass for the next five/seven years after menopause. However, if you are a fast bone loser, dropping 5 to 6 percent a year, you are at high risk for osteoporosis and your physician will strongly recommend hormone replacement.

This test is equally beneficial as a follow-up procedure. If you're not losing much bone right now, you may wish to wait and retest in a year or two when you see if the results warrant taking medication.

There are several different types of densitometry testing, but the most accurate is the dual-energy X-ray absorptiometry test (DEXA). The machine is generally available in most large hospitals in major cities and in dedicated menopause and osteoporosis clinics, and some physicians who treat arthritis and bone diseases may have the equipment right in their offices. The test is easy to take—you simply lie on a table as a picture is taken and relayed to a video screen across the room. It is noninvasive, and the machines emit a very small amount of radiation.

Q: If I'm concerned about heart disease, what tests would my physician order?
The doctor will check your blood pressure and heart rate, do routine blood tests (see above), and then perform an EKG to check for any abnormalities. If you have complained of chest pain or if the EKG has left any doubt as to your heart health, you will be sent to a cardiologist for an EKG/treadmill test, usually done in women with a radio-

active tracer such as thallium, to see how your heart performs under stress. A chest X-ray would be taken to see if you have any structural abnormalities or whether your heart is enlarged.

You might also have an echocardiogram to see how your heart valves are functioning and check the size of the four chambers of the heart.

If you have experienced any arrhythmias, your physician might ask you to wear a Holter monitor for twenty-four hours to make a continuous microchip recording of the heart's electrical activity.

If you have been having persistent angina (sharp chest pain), or suffer chest pains during your exercise stress test, your physician might order a cardiac catheterization to see if there are blockages in your coronary arteries. An EPS (electrophysiology study) is performed to check for the cause of persistent arrhythmias. This test is similar to a catheterization.

Other Types of Care: Menopause Clinics and Alternative Practitioners

Some women who feel that their physician is not truly dedicated to midlife practice may feel more comfortable at a menopause clinic, where all the patients are at about the same life stage with the same health concerns.

Still others feel that they do not wish to medicalize any aspect of their menopause, and yet are searching for good general health care at this time of life. There are many excellent practitioners of alternative therapies you may wish to consult. You can select other health practitioners whether or not you are also receiving conventional medical care.

Q: Will I get better care at a menopause clinic than with a private doctor?

The level of care depends on the clinic, just as it does with a private doctor. The benefit of visiting this type of facility is that the entire staff and all resources are devoted to the perimenopausal and postmenopausal woman.

Clinics are generally located within hospitals, most commonly teaching hospitals, and many have long waiting lists. You should know up front—and if they don't tell you, be sure to ask—whether this clinic is associated with a particular research project. You are not obliged to take a particular drug simply because it is the subject of investigation at this clinic. Be aware that your personal concerns may be given short shrift if in fact the goal of the clinic is to get as many participants in one study as it can.

There will be doctors, nurses, sex educators, and para-professionals on staff—you may not see the same people twice when you make your visits.

The advantage of being seen in a clinic is that you'll be able to get everything under one roof: physical exams, diagnostic tests and procedures, self-help information, educational seminars, psychological counseling, nutritional and exercise counseling, and possibly even stress management workshops.

Q: How can I find a practitioner if I don't want to take hormones and I'm interested in pursuing alternative therapies?

You should contact a naturopath, an osteopath, a family doctor who is interested in nutrition and supplemental vitamins, minerals, herbs, or a traditional Chinese or Ayurvedic physician if you are interested in those Eastern medical systems.

You can also see a conventional gynecologist to guide your health care who also feels comfortable about your seeing alternative health care providers. If you make it clear up front that you wish to maintain regular preventive care with this doctor, you should all be able to work together.

Q: How much can I self-treat with alternative therapies?

You won't go wrong with most therapies—you can use books, cassettes, and videotapes to gather enough information about diet, exercise, supplementation, stress management, acupressure, and homeopathy to make considerable changes in your health care.

Herbs, however, should be used *only* under the recommendation of a professional. Many are general tonics and will simply strengthen the body, but some are highly estrogenic and could cause problems in women predisposed to estrogen-dependent cancers. They should also not be used if you are on ERT or HRT.

It's also advisable to get professional help with certain types of mind-body treatments like biofeedback, yoga, tai chi chuan, Feldenkrais, Trager, or Alexander technique. You will be able to use these more safely and effectively after you have had a few classes.

Chapter Seven

Finding the Right Dosage and Regimen for You

Making the decision to begin hormone replacement therapy is a terribly difficult one for most women; but an even larger problem after choosing to start is figuring out how you're going to take your medication. There are so many ways of replacing hormones—you can swallow a pill or wear a patch; you can keep your period or try to avoid one if you like; you can take synthetic or natural medication; you can take a very low dosage or something slightly more potent, depending on your health status.

How do you make these decisions, and what will the consequences be? Can you change your mind once you've started on your regimen?

One of the primary issues in many women over fifty is whether they want to continue to bleed every month. Different regimens offer different options—the cyclic one gives you a "period" at the same defined time in your "cycle," whereas the combined continuous regimen should eliminate all bleeding—although breakthrough bleeding (bleeding unrelated to a regular period) may occur during the first six to nine months in many women.

Another issue has to do with our comfort or discomfort with synthetic drugs. Some products on the market, although altered in the laboratory so that they can be used in the human body, are "natural" because they come from animal and plant sources. There are conjugated equine estrogens in the oral dosage of HRT derived from horse urine, and the 17-beta estradiol in the transdermal patch is processed from phytosterols (estrogen look-alike molecules) in plants. However, the progesterone-like drugs known as progestins that have been used until fairly recently are synthetic and may cause unpleasant side effects in some women. Newer regimens use a natural progesterone made from soy or wild yams—and many people report that they respond better to this form of the medication.

Another question is whether the nonoral regimens (patch, gel, injection, or implant) are as effective as the tablet in terms of protection against heart disease and osteoporosis as well as relief of menopausal complaints. Some physicians are convinced that the oral regimen offers the most benefits—and, of course, there are more data to rely on for the oral forms because they were the first type on the market. However, other doctors are concerned about long-term use of any oral medication that may be responsible for increased risk of several serious illnesses, including breast cancer.

Naturally, you can only arrive at your own personal choice in consultation with your physician. It may take some fine-tuning to get the correct mix that alleviates symptoms, protects your heart and bones adequately, has minimal side effects, and also keeps you safe over the long run. By asking appropriate questions and working closely with your doctor, you'll be able to come up with the dosage and regimen suited to your particular needs.

The Regimens You Might Follow

There are a variety of different options for taking hormones. The following questions will detail the various possibilities so that you can choose the one that's right for you.

Q: What is a drug regimen?
A drug regimen specifies which drug you'll take, how often, and under what circumstances. In other words, your regimen might be to take estrogen (Premarin, 0.625 mg) once a day every day and a progestin (Provera, 2.5 mg) once a day every day. Certain regimens will require that you take a pill on an empty stomach or with meals, in the morning or evening, alone or in combination with other drugs.

Q: What are the various different ways of taking HRT?
All regimens of HRT include a progestin or natural progesterone along with estrogen:
Oral, combined continuous: Estrogen and a progestin or natural progesterone are taken daily. After the first six to nine months, your breakthrough bleeding may stop.
Oral, cyclic: Estrogen is given for the first twenty-five days of the month. A progestin or natural progesterone is added for days one to twelve or days twelve to twenty-five inclusive. You take no supplements for the remainder of the month and experience two or three days of light bleeding.
Oral, cyclic progestin and continuous estrogen: You take estrogen throughout the month; the progestin or natural progesterone for the last twelve to fourteen days of your cycle. Most women experience two to three days of light bleeding.
Patch: You may wear an estrogen transdermal patch on your hip or buttock, which you change every three days

or every seven days, depending on the product you use. You must apply the patch smoothly, allowing no bumps or bubbles, in order to get effective transmission of the estrogen into your system. The medication, contained in the plastic barrier, gets into your bloodstream directly through your skin, which acts as a semipermeable membrane.

Percutaneous gel: This estrogen gel is spread daily on the skin, including both arms, forearms, and shoulders. It dries in a couple of minutes and is absorbed completely.

Injection: This is not a preferred method of taking estrogen and would only be prescribed for a woman who has had a hysterectomy. Estrogen is delivered by a once-monthly injection, which enters the bloodstream directly. Because of the need for either regular doctor visits or self-administered injections, few physicians recommend it. It gives higher estrogen levels in the body that can taper off too quickly and is therefore not safe for a woman with an endometrium that might overgrow.

Subcutaneous implant: Similar to the Norplant contraceptive, this little pellet contains estrogen. It is set in place near the ovary and the hormone is slowly released into the bloodstream over a period of six months. Although common in Europe, the FDA has restricted the use of these pellets because there have been problems with removing them if a women has to go off hormone replacement due to some medical problem. This is not a common method of administration.

Estrogen cream: This cream is used only to alleviate vaginal dryness and painful intercourse. The usual administration is twice weekly, but not right before intercourse. It is not useful for alleviating other menopausal symptoms or protecting your heart and bones. Estrogen cream can be used without a progestin whether or not you still have a uterus—as long as you follow the instructions on the prescription and do not overuse the product. The low dosages prescribed do not give a concentration of estrogen strong enough to thicken the endometrium.

Other, less commonly used products:

The *vaginal ring* fits into the vagina like a diaphragm and emits estrogen in a timed-release fashion. It contains very small amounts of estrogen, not enough to be absorbed into the bloodstream, and is therefore useful for the treatment of vaginal dryness but not for protection against heart disease and osteoporosis.

Sublingual estrogen tablets (buccal estrogen) dissolve in the mouth and go from the mucous membranes into the bloodstream. This form of estrogen is apparently effective in relieving hot flashes.

Q: What are the various ways to take ERT?

All of the above regimens are also available for ERT, but, unlike HRT, you do not need to take a progestin or natural progesterone, since you have no uterus and therefore no endometrium to protect.

Q: Is the estrogen in the oral medications or patch the same estrogen I've been producing in my body?

No. The body produces three types of natural estrogen—estradiol, estrone, and estriol. The estrogen in oral Premarin is a conjugated equine estrogen, processed from horse urine. The estrogen in the Estraderm and Climara patches is 17-beta estradiol, processed from plant phytosterols.

Q: What are the most popular brand-name prescriptions for estrogen and estrogen plus progestin?

Estrogen, oral, cyclic, or continuous: Premarin is the most popular. The other commonly prescribed pills on the market are Estrace and Estratab.

Estrogen patch: The three-day Estraderm and seven-day Climara patches.

Estrogen cream: Premarin, Ogen, and Estrace all make a cream to be used in the vagina.

Oral estrogen combined with progestin: The new products Prempro and Premphase combine the estrogen and progestin in one pill. Prempro offers you a blister pack where you pop out one pill daily for a combined continuous dosage of both estrogen and progestin. The pill contains Premarin (conjugated equine estrogen) and Cycrin (medroxyprogesterone acetate tablets) and you take one a day, every day. For most women, monthly bleeding usually stops over the course of your first year on the medication.

If you prefer a cyclic regimen, you can take Premphase, also a single prescription product. This blister pack offers one estrogen pill for days one to thirteen, and one estrogen-plus-progestin pill for the last fourteen days of your cycle. In this regimen, you will experience monthly bleeding, as though you had a period.

Natural oral estrogens, cyclic or continuous: Ortho-Est is a more "natural" estrone product (processed from plant phytosterols like natural micronized progesterone), as is Ogen, manufactured by Upjohn and derived from wild yams. Tri-Est, a combination product using all three estrogens, is available from various pharmacies around the country and in Canada. These are the least commonly prescribed oral estrogens.

Q: Do doctors ever prescribe just the progestin, without estrogen?

Yes, actually, this is a fairly common practice with women in perimenopause who are bleeding heavily and irregularly and/or those who may have begun to have some menopausal complaints. The difficulties with periods are caused by anovulatory cycles (cycles where estrogen is produced without progesterone). In this case, most doctors either prescribe Provera in a 10 mg dose or natural micronized progesterone (three 100 mg capsules at bedtime because it tends to make you sleepy) for ten days of the month to bring on a period. There appears to be little risk of breast cancer with this therapy. You should have no PMS-type symptoms as you might in a combined regimen.

Some women at this time of life prefer to use just the ProGest cream to control menopausal symptoms. The cream can be applied daily to the hip or buttock.

Q: What are the various ways to take a progestin or natural progesterone?

Oral, synthetic: Provera or Cycrin (medroxyprogesterone acetate or MPA), 2.5 mg daily with combined continuous regimen, or 5 mg for the first or last two weeks of your cycle with cyclic regimen. A second type of progestin, Micronor (a 19-nor-steroid known as norethindrone), 0.7 mg daily, appears to be associated with fewer PMS symptoms than MPA. This progestin is derived from synthetic androgens.

IUD: For women in the perimenopause who may still need contraceptive protection, a Progestasert IUD is sometimes prescribed, which emits a small amount of a progestin over time. Some IUDs are good for a year; others for as many as six years.

Oral, natural: Natural micronized progesterone, 100 to 200 mg twice daily. This is a capsule in a peanut-oil base.

Cream, natural: Topical creams such as ProGest and Proganol, derived from wild yams and sold in health food stores (available without a prescription), are used by some women who choose not to take HRT but who want the beneficial effects of progesterone to alleviate some menopausal symptoms. These creams purport to contain 3 percent progesterone, a lower dosage than the capsule. Many pharmacies (see the Resource Guide, pages 224–226) will make up progesterone creams with 5 percent, 6 percent, or 10 percent progesterone. They also compound natural progesterone troches (which melt under the tongue) and vaginal suppositories.

Q: Why would any woman select the cyclic regimen, choosing to bleed when she doesn't have to?

For some, the sight of that monthly stain is a reassurance that everything is functioning well. Many women feel an affirmation of their femininity when they bleed. Also, it is easier to monitor something you can see than something you can't—you'll know that it's time to call your doctor if bleeding becomes excessive or stops entirely. Also, because most research has been done on the cyclic regimen, there is more scientific data to rely on in terms of safety and efficacy. Finally, there is no promise that you won't have some flow on the continuous regimen as well.

Q: How do I know that the bleeding I'm experiencing on HRT is normal?

If you're taking cyclic HRT (estrogen for days one to twenty-five and a progestin for twelve days) or continuous estrogen and cyclic progestin, you should expect several days of *withdrawal bleeding* when both hormones are withdrawn.

Irregular, midcycle bleeding, also known as *breakthrough bleeding*, may indicate that you need an adjusted dosage, or that your body has not yet adapted to its new schedule—or that you are bleeding for some other organic reason that should be investigated by your doctor.

If you are taking combined continuous HRT, where you take both hormones every day, you will probably continue to bleed for the first six to nine months of your therapy (and some women never stop). The farther away you are from your last menstrual period, the less likely you are to bleed on this regimen.

Q: Is it dangerous *not* to bleed once a month if you're taking estrogen?

The combined continuous regimen is safe even if you don't bleed. Although you don't slough off the old lining of the uterus, the endometrium stabilizes during the month from the hormonal stimulation it receives. The regular administration of estrogen and the progestin together each day ensures that the endometrium won't overgrow or develop cancerous cells.

Q: What's this I've heard about taking HRT with testosterone to improve my sex drive?

Females make testosterone just as males do (though they have about nine times less), and it is this hormone that triggers feelings of arousal and desire. At menopause, androgen levels can drop, resulting in a lowered libido.

If one of your menopausal problems is low sex drive, your physician may prescribe Estratest, an oral combination of estrogen and an androgen, or male gonadal hormone. Testosterone is combined with estrogen in this project to boost sexual interest. You can also take Premarin with methyltestosterone tablets (the oral form of testosterone). There are drawbacks to both oral and injectable testosterone. Testosterone has been shown to stimulate breast cancer cell division in the laboratory. A Danish study showed that women taking estrogen and testosterone together had twice the risk of breast cancer compared to those taking no medication.

Another risk associated with replacement testosterone is liver disease. There have been studies that show that very high doses of the oral form of testosterone (150 mg/day) can cause rare cases of hepatitis and liver cancer. (Lower dosages—1.25 to 10 mg daily—appear to be safe.)

The injectable form—testosterone enanthate—is generally given in dosages that may raise cholesterol levels and lower the good HDL cholesterol.

Probably the safest method of replacing testosterone is to apply a 1 percent cream of testosterone proprionate to the clitoris and surrounding area two or three times weekly. With oral and injectable forms of testosterone, if you have a uterus, you must also take a progestin or natural progesterone.

Q: Are there medications that can be combined with HRT to make me less depressed?

If you have been feeling depressed, and estrogen has not alleviated the problem, your physician may prescribe an antidepressant or mood stabilizer concurrent with your HRT. But just taking pills is never enough. Exercise is a big help because it encourages the production of beta endorphins, the natural opiates the brain makes that fill us with a sense of well-being. You may also consider a short course of psychotherapy with your medication and regular exercise. (See Chapter 9 for a full discussion of midlife and depression.)

Q: How much does HRT cost?

In most parts of the country, a yearly supply of estrogen (Premarin) costs from $170 to $200; an equivalent prescription of Tri-Est (1.25 mg twice daily) would cost $257. A yearly supply of progestin (Provera) would cost about $250; a roughly equivalent prescription of natural micronized progesterone (100 mg twice daily for the last fourteen days of your cycle) would cost about $220 a year, unless your physician wants you to take 300 mg instead of 200 mg daily for fourteen days, in which case you'd spend about $320 a year.

"Natural" or Synthetic Medication

Some drugs are processed from animal or plant sources; others are made in a laboratory. The "natural" products have been reported to cause fewer side effects; however, there are also fewer studies that can be cited on the efficacy of natural products. The following questions will explain the differences.

Q: Are some estrogen products more "natural" than others?

Certain naturopathic physicians prescribe Ortho-Est, Tri-Est, and Ogen instead of Premarin. (Ogen, made from wild yams, is the one that more doctors are likely to prescribe since it is manufactured by a major pharmaceutical company and the dosage is standardized.) These products use estrone sulfate instead of estradiol. Since estrone is the primary estrogen in a postmenopausal woman's body, Ortho-Est, Tri-Est, and Ogen are closer copies of what the body is actually manufacturing. Several pharmacies around the country will custom-compound estriol as well.

The transdermal patches (Estraderm, or the Climara seven-day patch) bypass the liver, and therefore carry no risk of gallbladder or liver disease. They also use 17-beta estradiol, from a plant source.

Q: What's the difference between the synthetic progestin and natural progesterone?

Synthetic progestins, also called *progestagens*, have long been the thorn in the side of proponents of HRT. Although these compounds mimic the action of progesterone, the body doesn't respond to it in the same way as it does to the natural variety. The problems of adding a progestin include unpleasant PMS-like side effects such as bloating, fatigue, mood swings, and tender breasts. There are also data that suggest an increased risk of breast cancer when a progestin is used.

Natural micronized progesterone is derived from a plant source—either a wild yam or a soybean plant phytosterol (a progesterone look-alike molecule) that has been altered in a laboratory so that it is more active and potent and can be well utilized in the human body. Initial experiments with this natural form had poor outcomes because a powdered form of the supplement was used, and progesterone in powder form is destroyed by stomach acids. But the new compound on the market is processed in an oil base that is absorbed first through the lymphatic system, and then passes through the liver to be metabolized.

The natural progesterone is more expensive, but many experts and women (who are the *real* experts) are so pleased with its results, they feel the extra cost is justified. Women who are taking natural progesterone experience fewer menopausal symptoms and those they do have are minor. The recent PEPI study (see Chapter 5) showed that use of natural micronized progesterone had the second most favorable results in terms of lipid levels after unopposed estrogen (synthetic progestins came in third). There have been no studies as yet on the effect of this "quasi" natural substance on bone density.

The only side effects that have been reported are some drowsiness and light-headedness when you first start the medication, but this soon passes, and the drug in general is much easier to tolerate than the synthetic variety.

Q: If micronized progesterone is so superior to the synthetic, why isn't every doctor recommending it?

The FDA has not yet approved a natural micronized progesterone product to be used in a hormone replacement therapy regimen. One major drug company is close to packaging a product that can be tested and therefore may be deemed acceptable, but in the meantime, you can only get natural micronized progesterone from a variety of pharmacies across the country who buy their raw product from some of the bigger pharmaceutical firms and compound their own brand.

Many physicians don't prescribe natural progesterone because there haven't yet been a lot of extensive clinical trials on it, and a dosage equivalent to synthetic progestin that will protect the endometrium is as yet uncertain. Although it appears to be superior in many ways to the synthetic progestin, it is not yet a well-known commodity.

With custom-compounding of a drug, there are marked differences in potency and batch-to-batch consistency. But with the recent serious scientific research that's been done using micronized progesterone, it's likely that the drug will be standardized and, within a year or two, a major pharmaceutical company will be selling it—which may make doctors feel more comfortable about recommending it. For pharmacies that will make up this product, see pages 224–226 in the Resource Guide.

You may have to ask your doctor to do some supplemental reading on this subject if you're interested in trying it.

Q: Would I take the natural progesterone the same way I take the synthetic?

No. Because "natural" medications have a shorter half-life than synthetic, it's important to take half your daily dose twice daily instead of the whole thing once daily, as you would with a synthetic.

Q: Since the synthetic progestin seems so problematic, is there any way for me to take *less* of this medication than is usually prescribed?

Certain physicians will allow you to take the progestin every other month or even every third month if you are carefully monitored. It has been shown that abnormal uterine lining cells begin to grow after only seventy-six days of unopposed estrogen—which means that it could be dangerous to skip more than two months of the progestin.

Many women so dislike the progestin part of the regimen because of its PMS-like side effects that they decide on their own to discontinue it while they take estrogen—but it must be stressed that this is a very wrongheaded idea for someone who still has her uterus.

Q: How will I know that the progestin is keeping my uterus healthy?

Your doctor will follow your bleeding pattern—which should be an indication of endometrial health. If you're bleeding irregularly, or are having a lot of breakthrough bleeding, he or she will want to check the inner lining and middle layer of your uterus—the endometrium and myometrium—for overgrowth or abnormal cells.

An endometrial biopsy, where a small piece of tissue is removed to analyze just the inner layer of the uterus, is the "gold standard" for diagnosis, although it is an invasive and uncomfortable procedure. Many physicians feel it should be done after several years on HRT, or if you are having unpredictable bleeding patterns on the medication.

Another possibility is to have a transvaginal ultrasound, using a probe inserted into the vagina. This is a more comfortable, noninvasive way to check the thickness of these two types of tissue.

Pill or Patch—What Are the Differences?

Some physicians prescribe oral medication because it offers relief from symptoms and confers long-term benefits, and others think that different forms of administration such as the patch, the gel, the injection, or an IUD are just as effective and may be safer. The answers to the following questions will explain the differences.

Q: What are the advantages of taking HRT orally?

The various different oral regimens have proven benefits for the heart and bones *in addition* to alleviating common problems of menopause such as hot flashes, vaginal dryness, mood swings, and sleep disturbances. In order for a medication to have maximum effect on all your body's organs, it must be ingested and metabolized. When you swallow a pill, the medication affects lipid levels as it works its way through the bloodstream, exerting its influence on the cardiovascular system, the musculoskeletal system, and the endocrine system. Estrogen keeps LDL cholesterol low and raises HDL cholesterol. It affects bone tissue by attaching to estrogen receptors on bone cells and retaining good mass and density.

Q: What are the disadvantages of the oral regimen?

Since all medication taken orally must pass through the gastrointestinal system and be delivered to the liver to be metabolized, there are rare cases where gallbladder or liver tumors develop. These tumors are usually benign, but still require medical or surgical care. Several other risks associated with estrogen use have to do with the production of proteins in the liver, which are not produced if you wear a patch or use the estrogen cream. (For a discussion of long-term safety on HRT, see Chapter 5.)

Also, many women are uneasy about taking a pill for something that is not a disease. Although it's true that all the various methods of administration deliver medicine just as a tablet does, the psychological effect of popping a pill every day is a liability for many individuals.

Q: What are the advantages and disadvantages of the patch?

A patch gets the medication right into the bloodstream, bypassing the liver. Early studies showed that the patch was beneficial for women at high risk for osteoporosis. It alleviates menopausal symptoms as well as the pill, if applied correctly and changed regularly.

Also, since you can see and feel a patch, it's easier to remember to change it than it is to take a pill every day. You're more likely to stick to your regimen if you have a good reminder.

One disadvantage of the patch is that you must apply it properly and be sure that it lies flat against your skin. If you do a lot of swimming or rub yourself roughly when you shower, and the patch starts coming off, you'll have to change it more frequently. Some women develop allergic reactions to the glue on the patches.

The major disadvantage of the patch is that it does not offer the same good lipid changes as the oral medication since it enters the bloodstream directly without being metabolized by the liver. In order to affect cholesterol levels, the drug needs this "first pass" in the liver, since one of the liver's functions is to manufacture and process cholesterol and deliver it into the bloodstream. For this reason, the patch is not recommended for women at high risk for heart disease.

Q: Why might my doctor prescribe an injection or an implant?

An injection is usually prescribed only for a woman who has had a hysterectomy and who has a lot of difficulty remembering a daily pill, has trouble applying the patch smoothly, or who needs supervision by her doctor to stay on target with her medication. This is not an advisable method of administering estrogen, and very few physicians will prescribe it. Because the injection causes much higher estrogen levels than any other method of administration, it is not recommended for a woman with an endometrium.

Implants, too, require little participation on the part of the patient, but very few doctors are currently prescribing them. The FDA has restricted their use because of concerns about removing them if patients develop medical problems that might prohibit use of estrogen.

Q: Why might my doctor prescribe an IUD with progestin in it?

For women who are perimenopausal and still have occasional periods on their own, but who do not choose to get pregnant again, this method of administration takes care of two problems at once—birth control and protection of the endometrium on an HRT regime.

The IUD dosage of progestin enters the bloodstream at the location where it's needed most, situated right next to the endometrium. For this reason, systemic risks and side effects should be minimal. Many physicians like to wean women off contraceptive birth control pills and onto a progestin at this time of life, and the IUD is a convenient way to do this for women who tolerate it well.

Some physicians are opposed to the use of IUDs in general, as they can cause increased pelvic inflammatory disease (PID), cramping, and bleeding, and if they fail in their contraceptive function, there can be dangers to the unborn child. The older forms of IUDs were made of metal, which often interacted badly with internal tissues. Today's IUDs, however, are made of inert materials (plastic or rubber) that are easier to wear.

Q: What if I am on oral hormones and forget to take my medication?

If you miss a day or two during the month, you probably won't notice a difference. If you skip too many days, you will upset the new hormonal balance that the medication is attempting to achieve and will probably have some breakthrough bleeding during the month. You may also experience a variety of menopausal symptoms such as hot flashes, vaginal dryness, mood swings, insomnia, and urinary incontinence.

It is more common that women "forget" the progestin and remember the estrogen—simply because they dislike the progestin's effects. But remember that the endometrium can overgrow within a few months if you don't take both medications. In order to make sure you get your appropriate medication, you may wish to try the two-pills-in-one regimens, Prempro or Premphase.

If you have problems remembering to take pills, you may do better with the patch (which you can *see* every time you take a shower or change your clothes), or the implant, which requires no maintenance and, if you have a uterus, the Progestasert IUD, which can remain in place for a year or more.

A Question of Dosage

Should you take little or a lot? Is it safer to start with the lowest dose and build up to a higher one? The following questions will help pinpoint the right dosage for you.

Q: How will my doctor decide what dosage is right for me?

The lower the dosage, the safer the regimen. The most common dosage of oral estrogen is 0.625 mg daily, which is the recommended amount to alleviate signs and symptoms of menopause and also protect your heart and bones.

For women who are only interested in short-term therapy, strictly to alleviate menopausal symptoms, many physicians will prescribe an even lower (0.3 mg) dosage, and if this does the job, it can be an extremely safe method of alleviating unpleasant symptoms. (It is probably not enough to give you the beneficial effects on your heart and bones unless you also exercise regularly, however.) For women who are not getting relief or who are at high risk for heart disease or osteoporosis, or who have had their ovaries removed, the physician may wish to prescribe a higher dosage (0.9, 1.25, 2.5 mg).

It is important to note that an increased incidence of breast cancer has only been noted in dosages above 0.625, which means that it's important to discuss your desire to stick to a low dosage with your doctor.

The dosage of the patch is calculated differently from that of the pill because the type of estrogen used is different. Each three-day patch contains either 0.05 mg or 0.1 mg of 17-beta estradiol. There are also seven-day patches that can deliver a similar amount of estrogen, and you don't have to remember to change them as often.

Estrogen creams contain 0.625 mg per gram (Premarin cream) or 0.1 mg of 17-beta estradiol per gram (Estrace cream).

The dosage of progestin depends on whether you're on combined continuous regimen, i.e., taking it daily (in which case it's usually 2.5 mg of Provera or an equivalent progestin), or on the cyclic regimen for just two weeks a month (in which case it's usually 5 mg Provera). If you are taking natural micronized progesterone, the dosage is most commonly 75 to 100 mg twice daily, or, on a cyclic regimen, from 100 to 300 mg a day for ten days. It should be noted that the amount needed to protect the endometrium has not yet been established.

Length of Treatment, Contraindications, and Stopping Treatment

The decisions you make about HRT should be based on your general health and your reasons for taking the medication in the first place. It's important to ask questions about any conditions that would prevent you from taking this therapy, how long you should be on it, and how to stop if you decide it's not for you. See Chapter 5 for all questions about risks and side effects.

Q: How long do I have to be on HRT?

It depends on your purpose. If you are interested only in relief of unpleasant symptoms, such as alleviating hot flashes and vaginal dryness, restoring your interest and enjoyment of sex, sleeping soundly, and leveling out mood swings or depression, then you probably need to take this medication only as long as these problems persist. For most women, the intensity of menopausal complaints lasts less than five years. (Vaginal dryness, which can persist into extreme old age, can generally be handled with natural lubricants.)

However, if you are at high risk for osteoporosis or heart disease, there is really no limit to the length of your therapy. LTHRT (long-term HRT) could be lifelong for many women.

But because there are no studies that go out further than fifteen years, you can't rely on firm scientific data when making your decision to stay on HRT for longer. This is a matter you'll have to consider seriously.

Q: Why would I be told that I should not take *any* HRT regimen?

Anyone with a history of estrogen-dependent breast or uterine cancer is advised not to take HRT. Other conditions that could make HRT inadvisable or prohibited (depending on your physician's opinion) would be undiagnosed abnormal genital bleeding; an active or past history of problems with blood clots; stroke; liver dysfunction or disease; gallbladder or kidney dysfunction or disease; or asthma, epilepsy, or migraines.

Q: If I decide that I don't like taking HRT, can I stop cold turkey?

You should discuss your concerns with your physician and let him or her guide you as you taper off the medication slowly. He or she may counsel you to go from one estrogen tablet a day (on oral medication) to one every other day for a month, then twice weekly for another month, and finally, one a week for a few more weeks before stopping. Don't cut back on the progestin or natural progesterone while you're tapering off estrogen—continue your regular dosage until the very end, when you can stop it completely.

If you're wearing the patch, you should cut each one in half, tape the edges, and continue using it that way for a month, changing it once a week or twice a week depending on your dosage, after which time you can stop.

Q: What happens to my body when I stop taking HRT?

Stopping abruptly may bring on a rash of menopausal complaints such as hot flashes, vaginal dryness, and unusual bleeding patterns.

In addition, studies have shown that stopping HRT immediately causes a setback in good bone maintenance, and whatever mass and density have been preserved by taking HRT are soon lost. It's also evident that you can't retain the lipid levels and vascular elasticity that you've gained on the medication.

However, if you continue to exercise and begin to substitute natural treatments for the medication, you can improve your overall good health and do a great deal to protect yourself against future degenerative diseases.

Complementary Natural Treatments

HRT isn't the only consideration you have at midlife. To stay healthy or get healthy, and to relieve menopausal symptoms, you should also think about natural remedies and treatments. See also Chapters 3 and 10 to learn more about alternative and complementary treatments and remedies that you can use for menopausal complaints.

Q: Which natural treatments can I combine with HRT or ERT?

With very few exceptions, natural therapies are wonderful adjuncts to HRT. It's clear that diet and exercise, vitamin and mineral supplementation (particularly vitamin E for hot flashes and your heart and calcium for your bones), homeopathy, many herbs, cognitive-behavioral therapy, bodywork therapies, and stress management techniques such as meditation, visualization, yoga, tai chi chuan, acupuncture, and biofeedback can help *everyone*, whether or not they decide to take medication. They all provide a healthier body and immune system, which means that you can withstand the aging process better than you could without them.

Q: Are there any natural remedies that should not be combined with HRT or ERT?

Some herbs are estrogenic, that is, they contain the same active ingredients as HRT or ERT. Ginseng, false unicorn, blessed thistle, wild yam root, dong quai/dang gui, and black cohosh should not be combined with your medication. This is also true of the supplement evening primrose oil.

If you are working with a traditional Chinese or Ayurvedic (Indian) medical practitioner, he or she too would probably advise against HRT because of chemical interference with many herbs and treatments used in their work.

Chapter Eight

Dealing with Hysterectomy and Oophorectomy

Next to the C-section, the most performed operation in the United States is the hysterectomy, or surgical excision of the uterus and cervix. Oophorectomy, removal of the ovaries, is an even more radical procedure. Nearly 600,000 American women a year undergo hysterectomy; of these, nearly 480,000 undergo oophorectomy.

In about 10 percent of cases, these procedures are absolutely essential and save lives. In about 90 percent of cases, however, the surgery is elective and is performed, one would hope, to improve the quality of life. But many—some say most—of these procedures may be unnecessary. Thousands of hysterectomies are performed for lack of confidence on the part of the physician and patient that there is any other alternative. Years ago, many physicians routinely recommended hysterectomy to any woman in midlife who came in complaining of irregular bleeding or any chronic menopausal discomfort. And although today the medical community is more enlightened, far too many women are losing reproductive organs—not to mention crucial hormonal stimulation.

The decision to take hormones is pretty well made for you if you have one of these procedures, since your own hormonal production is radically changed by the surgeries. Hysterectomy may speed up menopause by about five years because blood flow to the estrogen-producing ovaries is jeopardized, which means that you may have that many more years of bone loss and of lack of estrogen protection to the heart. A hysterectomy prior to menopause greatly increases the risk of developing heart disease. When the ovaries are removed as well, you immediately lose the source of your hormonal production, which can mean a severe and dramatic series of menopausal complaints in addition to increased risk for osteoporosis and heart disease.

In this chapter, we'll answer questions relevant to the procedures themselves and also to the burning desire on the part of most women to save their reproductive organs.

All About Hysterectomy

Q: What is a hysterectomy?
A hysterectomy may be either subtotal, where only the uterus is removed, or total, where both your uterus and its lower end, or cervix, are removed. Afterward, your ovaries will continue to produce estrogen and progesterone, but you will not bleed since you won't have an endometrium (the lining of the uterus that is sloughed off each month in response to hormonal fluctuations). Since you have no place for an egg to implant, you can't get pregnant, either.

Q: At what age are most hysterectomies performed?
Most women who undergo this procedure are under forty-five.

Q: What are some symptoms for which a hysterectomy might be recommended?

A hysterectomy might be recommended if your Pap test indicates an abnormality; if you have dysfunctional (and debilitating) bleeding; if you have severe, unexplained pelvic pain; if your bowel or bladder isn't functioning as it should; or if your doctor can feel a mass during a physical exam or see a mass on an ultrasound test. Unless the mass is found to be cancerous, none of these is a definite indication that a hysterectomy is necessary.

Q: What are the most common reasons given for doing a hysterectomy?

The most common reasons are fibroids that cause abnormal bleeding or are pressing on other organs, uterine prolapse, adenomyosis, or cervical or endometrial cancer.

Q: My doctor is concerned about my abnormal bleeding patterns. Am I going to need a hysterectomy?

A hysterectomy should be the last resort to stop bleeding. During the perimenopause, it's common to have very long cycles (every eighty to ninety days) and very short cycles (every ten to fifteen days) or anywhere in between. Perimenopausal women tend to flow more heavily because their estrogen levels are higher before ovulation and lower after ovulation—or they may have anovulatory cycles, which also tend to produce a heavier flow and a more irregular cycle.

Q: What are fibroids?

Fibroids are growths of tissue, usually benign, that originate in the uterine muscle. As long as they stay the same size, no treatment is necessary. But if they start growing, which most do under the influence of estrogen, they can cause bleeding and pressure on other organs, which may cause constipation, incontinence, or bladder problems that may lead to kidney damage. However, it may be possible to remove the fibroids without removing the uterus.

Q: What is uterine prolapse?

With age, or many pregnancies, many women begin to experience a weakening of the pelvic floor muscles. Over time, the uterus may collapse so far into the vaginal canal that the cervix comes through the vaginal opening or the entire uterus drops down through the vagina.

In order to conserve the uterus of a premenopausal woman who may want more children, many doctors will try uterine suspension surgery, in which the ligaments that hold up the uterus are tightened and shortened. This works in some cases; in others, the ligaments stretch and the surgery must be repeated. Some physicians recommend a pessary, a rubber stopper that fits around the cervix, to hold the organs in place.

A very fit postmenopausal woman might be given a uterine suspension, where the ligaments that have stretched out are surgically shortened and lifted. However, most physicians recommend hysterectomy for uterine prolapse in postmenopausal women, since stop-gap measures usually don't work and may require repeated surgeries.

Q: Is there any way to prevent uterine prolapse?

The best preventive treatment is doing daily Kegel exercises. In order to do a Kegel, pretend that you are sitting on the toilet releasing a stream of urine. Now contract the muscles around the urethra and vagina and stop the stream. That is one Kegel. They can be done quickly or slowly to strengthen these muscles. Try three sets of ten, three times a day. You may also be told to exercise with weighted vaginal cones, holding a weight of several ounces in the vagina for fifteen minutes twice daily. There are five different weights—and just as you'd do with your Nautilus training, you work your way from the lightest to the heaviest. (See the Resource Guide, page 224.)

Q: What is adenomyosis?

In this condition, usually found in older premenopausal women, cells from the lining of the uterus migrate to the uterine muscle walls, which then become enlarged and tender, particularly when engorged with blood during a period.

Since this condition usually improves after menopause (when the ebb and flow of hormones cease), most physicians are very conservative about recommending hysterectomy for adenomyosis. However, this condition may predispose you to future cancer of the uterus, so it is crucial that you are carefully monitored. If the condition worsens, hysterectomy will be recommended.

Q: Are endometrial and cervical cancers life-threatening, and will I need a hysterectomy to cure them?

Experts often refer to these as the "good" cancers (if there can be such a thing) because they can be easily detected and cured in their early stages. Hysterectomy is warranted only in cases that haven't responded to other types of therapy or cancers that are not diagnosed until they are in advanced stages.

Cervical cancer is detected by a Pap smear and a colposcopy, where a group of cells is taken from the cervix, stained, and examined under a high-power microscope. This type of cancer is usually treated by removing a cone-shaped wedge of cancerous cells by laser surgery or by LEEP (loop electrosurgical excision procedure).

Endometrial cancer is detected and often treated with a D&C (dilatation and curettage). The cervix is dilated so that a thin instrument can be inserted into the uterus to scrape off the endometrium. The resulting tissue will be examined for cancerous cells. If such cells are present, your doctor may recommend a hysterectomy. Less radical procedures used to treat this condition (depending on the stage in which it's detected) are endometrial ablation (a laser procedure), or resectoscopic surgery (partial excision of the endometrium) using the hysteroscope.

Q: How would my doctor know that I had endometrial cancer and would a hysterectomy cure it?

This cancer is detected by a biopsy or D&C. Some surgeons recommend chemotherapy or radiation therapy, and a hysterectomy is recommended only if the cancer is not detected until it is in a very advanced stage.

Q: What is an oophorectomy?

An oophorectomy is surgery to remove the ovaries, which produce estrogen and progesterone. If your uterus is not diseased, it is not removed in this procedure. However, when there is a problem with all the organs, and the uterus, cervix, fallopian tubes, and ovaries must be removed, this is known as a *total abdominal hysterectomy and bilateral salpingo-oophorectomy* (TAHBSO).

An oophorectomy is often called "female castration" because your source of hormonal production is gone for good. You are no longer able to bear children and will also go through menopause rapidly after this surgery, which means that you will become at higher risk for heart disease and osteoporosis.

Q: Why would my doctor feel I needed this drastic procedure?

The most common reasons for oophorectomy are a tumor on the ovary that is suspected to be malignant, ovarian or other estrogen-dependent cancer, or chronic and severe endometriosis.

Q: How would my doctor know that I had ovarian cancer, and is there anything that could prevent it?

Cancer of the ovaries is the most difficult cancer to detect; unfortunately, there are usually no symptoms until the disease is in its advanced stages. Oophorectomy followed by radiation is the recommendation for most cases. Although little is known about this cancer, it seems that having taken birth control pills during your reproductive years is protective against it.

Q: Is an oophorectomy always necessary after breast cancer?

Your physician may feel that this is a prudent choice, since breast cancer proliferates under the influence of estrogen. This is especially true if you had one mastectomy, and then, several years later, had a recurrence of the cancer in the other breast.

However, it is also possible that if you have undergone chemotherapy or radiation therapy, your ovaries may no longer be producing estrogen—and therefore you would not need surgery. A blood test would confirm your current level of circulating estrogens.

Q: What is endometriosis?

In this disease, cells from the endometrial lining implant themselves on other organs in the pelvic cavity where they grow and proliferate, causing pain and often preventing proper functioning of bowel and bladder. Some cases can be handled with medication (GnRH agonists such as Lupron, or a synthetic androgenic compound, Danazol) and laser surgery; however, some resistant cases may require an oophorectomy to remove the estrogen source.

Alternatives to Hysterectomy and Oophorectomy

Hysterectomy and oophorectomy are radical surgical procedures, and if they can be safely avoided, they should be. You'll need at least two professional opinions before you'll know whether your ultimate health depends on losing or keeping these organs.

Heavy bleeding can often be checked by D&Cs, endometrial ablation, and heat ablation; myomectomy can be used for many fibroids; and hormones can be given to a patient with fibroids or overgrowth of the endometrium that causes bleeding but is not cancerous.

Q: I have fibroids, but I'm not really bleeding a lot and they don't make me too uncomfortable. Do I need a hysterectomy?

Every case is different. If your uterus is packed with many fibroids, you may need some surgery, but it's conceivable that your doctor could remove the fibroids and leave your uterus intact—a procedure called a *myomectomy*. Or your physician may advise that you wait for menopause, when the fibroids will shrink due to lack of estrogen stimulation.

Q: Would a D&C be an alternative if I'm bleeding a lot?

It might be. A dilatation and curettage (D&C) is a diagnostic procedure to discover the cause of abnormal bleeding. However, the procedure itself may stop the bleeding. Some of the extracted tissue will be examined under a high-power microscope for uterine cancer, hyperplasia (overgrowth) of the endometrium, or polyps.

Q: What is endometrial ablation, and is it an alternative?

The procedure known as endometrial ablation is an alternative to hysterectomy. In this type of surgery, the endometrium, or lining of the uterus, is destroyed with a laser. A thin probe called a hysteroscope is inserted through the cervix. The uterus is then pumped with carbon dioxide so that the surgeon can view the entire interior of the organ through lenses. Using another tube with a laser on the end, the surgeon then destroys the endometrium. After the procedure, you will have no period (since the layer of cells that replenish the lining of the uterus has been obliterated with the laser). This procedure also renders you sterile, because the tissue is inhospitable to supporting an egg that might implant.

Q: What is a heat ablation?

A balloon is inserted past the cervix into the uterus and filled with a sterile solution until it conforms to the shape of the interior of the uterus. A heating element then raises the temperature of the solution to 189 degrees Fahrenheit, permanently destroying the endometrium. Finally, the balloon is withdrawn.

Of the women who've undergone this procedure so far, 25 to 30 percent stopped bleeding entirely and a full 50 percent had a reduced flow.

This type of ablation, currently being tested in several U.S. hospitals, also causes sterility.

Q: Can I take hormone therapy to reduce my fibroids?

Yes, but HRT isn't the regimen that's used. Oral contraceptives and progestins are used, as well as gonadotropin releasing hormones (GnRH). The GnRH agonists Lupron and Synarel stop your period. These drugs may bring on menopausal symptoms such as hot flashes, vaginal dryness, and reduced bone mass and density. Because long-term use of these drugs can be severely detrimental to your bone health, many doctors will use them to shrink tumors prior to myomectomy or may use them to buy time until menopause, when declining estrogen levels will cause the tumors to reduce in size and/or vanish.

Q: What is a myomectomy, and how is it used for fibroids?

In this surgical procedure, the fibroids are removed one at a time from the uterus through an abdominal incision (although small or conveniently located fibroids may be removed vaginally with an instrument called a hystero-scope). You are a good candidate for this procedure only if you have a few fibroids. Since fibroids are fed by estrogen, many of them regrow, and a quarter of women who've had this procedure have to have it again. However, a myomectomy does preserve the uterus, and if you can keep this vital organ until menopause (when your estrogen production declines), you may never need a hysterectomy.

Testing to Determine Whether You Need a Hysterectomy or Oophorectomy

In order to be absolutely certain that surgery is the correct choice in your particular situation, you will have several diagnostic tests.

Q: What tests would my doctor perform to see if I needed one of these procedures?

The following procedures will help your physician find out what might be wrong:

Vaginal ultrasound (to check the thickness of the vaginal tissue and endometrium): This noninvasive test involves placing a probe high up in the vaginal barrel that is connected to an ultrasound machine, which uses radio waves to measure the thickness of the tissue. A transducer wand is passed over the area and a picture and measurements are visible on a monitor.

D&C (to discover the cause of abnormal bleeding): See page 36 for a description of this procedure.

Endometrial aspiration (to detect endometrial cancer or overgrowth of endometrial cells): The cervix is dilated so that a hollow tube can be inserted; at this point, endometrial cells are sucked out for examination. This is an office procedure.

Hysteroscopy, endometrial biopsy (to detect abnormalities of the uterine cavity such as fibroids, polyps, or uterine cancer): The cervix is dilated to allow passage of a telescopelike instrument with an attachment on the end that can extract a sample of cells for examination.

Colposcopy, cervical biopsy, cone biopsy (to detect abnormalities of the cervix): Various surgical instruments are used to take cells from the cervix for examination.

What If You Really Do Need Surgery?

If your tests are positive, or if alternative treatments are not viable in your case, you will have to have the surgery. There are many important questions you should ask so that you'll be able to prepare ahead of time to get the best possible care.

Q: Will the surgeon I've consulted do the surgery, or will he have his residents do it?

Don't be embarrassed—always ask your doctor! If you are under the care of a very prestigious physician, he or she may in fact ask assistants to do the brunt of the work.

This is not necessarily a bad thing—newly trained doctors working under the direction of a surgical chief have to be expert at what they do, and they're willing and eager to get more surgical experience.

Q: Should I have blood drawn in case I need a transfusion?

It is highly unlikely that you would need blood during these procedures. However, if you will feel more comfortable knowing that you are prepared for anything, arrange to donate a week prior to your surgery. The blood is good—only for you, since it hasn't been tested for donation—for thirty-five days, in case of complications following your surgery.

Q: How long will I be in the hospital?

The usual stay for either hysterectomy or oophorectomy is three to four days, unless you have complications from surgery.

Q: What are the risks of having my uterus and/or ovaries removed?

When you take any organ out of the body, you are losing part of the entire system's function. Since the ovaries get part of their blood supply from arteries that branch out of the uterus and these are removed during a hysterectomy, blood (and the hormones that travel in the blood) isn't as available to the ovaries after a hysterectomy. Hysterectomized women have lower estrogen and progesterone levels and higher FSH and LH levels than women with intact uteruses.

If you have had your ovaries removed as well as your uterus, you no longer produce those hormones that interact with blood and bone cells. After an oophorectomy, you are at an even greater risk than after hysterectomy of both heart disease and osteoporosis.

Although you do not need your uterus for a pregnancy after menopause, it may be a component of your sexual responsiveness, and it holds a place in your pelvic cavity. Without a uterus, organs in the pelvic cavity shift and change place—which can lead to disruption in function.

Another risk of these surgeries is undergoing anesthesia. The lungs are always slightly compromised after having taken in these chemicals.

Q: Is there any way to keep producing estrogen after my ovaries are removed so that I won't have an instant menopause?

Depending on your condition, your doctor may feel that it will be safe to leave a portion of an ovary if it is not diseased. Even a small piece may continue to function normally, giving you a reasonable supply of hormonal stimulation.

All women produce a weaker form of estrogen, called estrone. The adrenals are responsible for putting out a male sex hormone called androstenedione, which after menopause is converted by the body's fat cells into estrone. Women who carry a little more weight, and therefore have more fat cells, produce more estrone.

What Should I Do and How Will I Feel After Surgery?

Having these organs removed makes the hormone decision easier because you will need more estrogen for a longer period of time than you would have had you gone through a natural menopause. This is a crucial time for you—the sooner you start feeling like your old self again and making some new accommodations to your new self, the better.

Q: After these surgeries, should I be taking hormone replacement?

ERT (estrogen replacement therapy) is almost always recommended for women who have had an oophorectomy. After this procedure, the hormonal system is like an electrical current with no outlet—although the brain continues to produce hormones, they no longer trigger production of gonadal hormones (estrogen and progesterone) in the reproductive system. Consequently, a sudden onset of hot flashes, vaginal dryness, joint pain, headaches, and other menopausal problems can cause you to feel miserable and fatigued. Also, without your gonadal hormones, you are instantly at higher risk for osteoporosis and heart disease.

ERT can also be helpful for women who have had hysterectomies. Even though their ovaries are still putting out some hormones, the arteries that join the ovaries to the uterus have been cut during surgery, and the hormonal supply is no longer as available to the rest of the bloodstream.

The benefit of having a hysterectomy is that, since you have no uterus and therefore no endometrial lining that could overgrow, you don't need a progestin. The progestin part of HRT is the one that is most problematic, since it raises LDL levels, and also produces uncomfortable PMS symptoms, so the therapy is more beneficial and far more palatable to most women.

Q: How long will it take me to feel fully functional again?

It usually takes at least six weeks to recover physically—this is major surgery—and you shouldn't be surprised if it takes a few months. If your procedure was done through an incision in your abdomen, you will have a sore stomach and pelvic area and find it difficult to stretch or walk briskly. Under no circumstances should you do any lifting—even making a bed—for four weeks, and you shouldn't do any heavy work for six to eight weeks postoperatively. At your six-week checkup, your physician can give you the go-ahead to do some easy exercises so that you can start to get back in shape.

A procedure done with a vaginal incision is easier to recover from, but you will have a higher risk of running a fever and getting a urinary tract infection (since you will have been catheterized during the surgery) and will probably need antibiotics during your recovery. The vaginal hysterectomy may interfere with G-spot stimulation during sex and may also prevent the "ballooning" of the vagina that occurs before orgasm to enhance pleasure.

You may have complications with the surrounding organs. Urinating may feel different now that your bladder is no longer connected to a uterus. You may have a temporary retention or incontinence problem; doing your Kegels daily will allow you to recover fully. You may also have a "lazy bowel" for several days after surgery, but stool softeners and increased fiber will get your bowel function back again.

Q: Should I stay in bed when I get home, and for how long?

It shouldn't be necessary to spend the day in bed, but it's important that you get sufficient rest after any major surgery. When you feel tired, get off your feet or even take a nap. If you overdo, you will not only feel awful; you also run the risk of a longer recuperation.

Prior to your surgery, make sure you have arranged for people to take over some of your more difficult chores. If you live alone, you'll want to set up a relief squad of friends and relatives who can drive you around or do a little light shopping for you if necessary.

Q: When can I have intercourse again?

Most physicians ask you to wait until your six-week post-operative check, but some women feel uncomfortable with anything inside the vagina for three to four months. (The vaginal barrel temporarily shrinks after the surgery—as more blood supply gets to the area over time, it becomes more elastic again.)

You can engage in all kinds of nonpenetrative sex as soon as you feel up to it. Hugging and kissing will do a lot to get you back on the road to enjoying your sexuality again.

Q: How soon will I be able to get back to work?

This is entirely an individual decision and will be based on the type of work you do and how you feel. You should plan to take two to three weeks off from your office. If you work at home, try to do a little more each day. If you do any kind of physical work, or have to be on your feet a lot, you will probably not be fully functional for six weeks after your surgery. You should get your physician's okay even before starting back part-time.

Q: Are there natural remedies I should be taking after a hysterectomy?

It's a good idea to get your diet and exercise regimes under strict control. Many women gain weight after surgical menopause, not because losing the reproductive organs puts on pounds, but because they have lost their interest in staying healthy, fit, and attractive.

Diet: A well-rounded, low-fat, high-carbohydrate diet that is primarily made up of whole grains, vegetables, fruits, and legumes, with some fish and skinned poultry several times a week, is a wonderful choice for any midlife woman, particularly after surgery. Be sure you are eating a lot of fiber, which not only improves bowel function, but reduces LDL cholesterol.

Supplementation: After these surgeries, it is important to take daily calcium (1,000 mg if you are on ERT or HRT, or 1,500 mg if you're not taking ERT or HRT) and magnesium (500 to 750 mg) and make sure you have enough vitamins B_6 (100 mg daily), C (500 to 1,000 mg daily), and E (400 to 800 IU daily) and zinc (15 mg). Right after surgery, when you have increased need for hemoglobin, you also may wish to supplement iron (which is included in most multivitamins). If you're getting 50 mg daily, that's sufficient.

Exercise: Exercise is one of the best gifts you can give yourself after a hysterectomy or oophorectomy. Starting with gentle stretches and warmups after your surgery—only after your doctor gives you the go-ahead—you should proceed to a full-fledged activity schedule every day. Start with your Kegels (see page 182 for a full description) in order to get your pelvic floor muscles back in shape.

Exercise offers innumerable benefits:

First, it stimulates the production of beta endorphins in the brain, those natural opiates that block pain and give us a sense of well-being.

Next, weight-bearing exercise (any activity that makes you work your body's weight against gravity) is the best natural bone-builder available. Since you are at higher risk for osteoporosis after these surgeries, you need a supplemental source of bone strength, and exercise provides that. You can also increase your cardiovascular health with aerobic exercise, which means you can decrease your risk of heart disease. Finally, exercise burns calories and motivates you to stick with good, healthy eating.

Herbal remedies: Prior to surgery, take 25 drops of tincture of echinacea root one to three times daily to speed healing.

Motherwort and chaste tree will add thickness to vaginal walls.

Homeopathy: Take belladonna, bryonia, or lycopodium for a painful, dry vagina. Sepia is also recommended for vaginal problems.

Sitz baths: Put about three or four inches of warm water in the bathtub or in a bidet or basin. You can make up an infusion of comfrey root (also known as "knitbone") and add that to the water.

Massage: One of the best things you can do for yourself is have a professional massage once a week after your surgery (and you can keep this up as long as you like—or let your partner take over if it becomes too expensive). Massage helps to stimulate the flow of hormones and will also restore energy to a body that is recovering from surgery. A professional will know just how much pressure to exert in various areas.

Q: Will a hysterectomy or oophorectomy make me feel less feminine?

It shouldn't, yet many women say that it does. The womb is traditionally the symbol of women's fecundity and reproductive ability. The ovaries, of course, are the primary organs that confer female gender. Although the outside world can never know that you have lost these organs, the thought of being without the trappings of your femininity can cause great psychic damage postoperatively.

It is important that you understand that your attractiveness is not based in your physical structure, but rather in your personality, your intellect, and your spirit. After hysterectomy, the quality of your orgasm may change significantly, and after oophorectomy, your libido may vanish completely. About half of all women who undergo this surgery say that they are no longer interested in sex—although this could be a compounded problem from a long recovery with internal adhesions and a vagina that feels bruised and sore. The longer you don't have intercourse, the less you feel you want to try it.

There are numerous studies that indicate that hysterectomy increases the risk of depression within three years of surgery. However, other studies show that women were happier when the source of pain and bleeding was removed. Being informed and prepared for surgery may make the difference.

Q: I've had a hysterectomy, and sex doesn't feel the same. Why is this?

Although a hysterectomy doesn't show the way a breast excision does, it also symbolizes the obliteration of part of the "woman" in you. If you no longer have a uterus, or a uterus and ovaries, you may feel neutered and therefore less sexual.

True, it's the vagina and not the uterus that receives the penis during intercourse; however, many women claim that the experience isn't as pleasurable after a hysterectomy. They're not just imagining that they've lost an integral part of their sexual equipment—in fact, they have. The uterus, far from being simply a bag to hold a baby, is a functional organ. It produces beta endorphins within the glands of the endometrium (those neurotransmitters that help to make us feel good), and the nerve endings at the cervical tip respond to deep thrusting during intercourse. Cervical mucus, produced at the tip of the uterus, helps with lubrication. The uterus also lifts and throbs during orgasm. So it's understandable that without all these advantages, sex might not feel as enjoyable.

It's important to ask your surgeon to shorten the vagina as little as possible, so that you can accommodate a penis of any length. If you are feeling less desire, the reason may be because of a decrease in circulating androgens (testosterone) that takes place when your ovaries are removed along with your uterus, so supplementing estrogen with testosterone may be a solution (see Chapter 7).

Q: Who can I talk to who will understand what I'm going through?

Sometimes you need a friend. As statistics show you, you have many, many friends out there who have gone through exactly what you are now experiencing. There are hundreds of support groups around the country, and by calling around to various women's organizations and hospitals, you will probably find one right near you.

Short-term psychotherapy may be helpful if you are struggling with a variety of issues surrounding your hysterectomy. If you find yourself feeling hopeless, sexless, or too confused to think straight, contact a therapist or social worker. Your physician or local women's center can give you a recommendation to a licensed professional.

For help in locating support groups, licensed professionals, national organizations, and medical information, see the Resource Guide, pages 213–224.

Chapter Nine

Exciting New Developments in the Use of Estrogen

It is clear that life can be made better for many women by helping them prevent disease conditions from developing. Estrogen is not only beneficial for the prevention of osteoporosis and heart disease and the relief of menopausal signs and signals—it also has potential to help those with other chronic conditions.

This hormone is quite likely to offer numerous advantages to those who suffer from problems with sexuality to urinary incontinence, Alzheimer's disease, and clinical depression. Although the benefits are not yet as certain as those for osteoporosis and heart disease, early studies look promising, and more information about the use of this hormone for these conditions is coming out each day.

Sexuality at midlife can be problematic for some women who experience a loss of desire or physical problems such as vaginal dryness or pain. Vaginal atrophy—the decline of the vagina and surrounding organs—and a loss of lubrication can certainly interfere with sexual delight. But HRT or ERT, as well as herbal remedies, can revitalize your sex life.

Urinary incontinence, where the bladder cannot hold urine, is a humiliating condition that often hits in midlife and impairs social interaction as well as physical function. Estrogen has been found to impart great benefits to some women with this problem.

There are also promising hints about using estrogen replacement for women with Alzheimer's disease, a condition that destroys the fabric of life as it erodes the cortex of the brain.

Depression is only partly triggered by hormones: we know that there are many factors—physical, mental, emotional, and social—that contribute to a feeling of despondency and hopelessness. But interesting work with HRT has shown that some women do respond very well to supplemental estrogen at this time of life.

Questions About Sexuality

Estrogen is great nourishment for the vagina, vulva, and uterus. Whether you choose to take the oral regimen, wear the patch, or just wish to use the cream topically, you will see relief of sexual discomfort quickly with HRT or ERT.

Q: What will HRT do for my sex life?
Estrogen affects more than three hundred tissues in the body, one of which is the brain—which helps you with the desire to engage in sexual activity in the first place. Of course, HRT also improves vaginal acidity levels and increases fluid and blood flow to the genitals. It plumps out the labia, adds layers of epithelial cells to the mucous membranes, and makes sure that the uterus does not collapse forward or backward in the pelvic cavity. Estrogen facilitates vaginal lubrication and generally keeps you free from irritation and infection. It helps to prevent inconti-

nence by strengthening the musculature around the urethra. Estrogen, of course, is also beneficial to the heart, which should be in good shape so that you feel energetic and healthy enough for sex.

But if the only midlife complaint you have is vaginal dryness, and it makes you too uncomfortable to enjoy sex, try the estrogen cream first, to see if this is sufficient medication for you. The topical cream plumps up the tissues and makes them less friable—which means that they can be rubbed or pinched or stroked without causing pain. It allows the vaginal tissues to lubricate when you are aroused, which heightens pleasure, and also allows comfortable penetration of a finger, penis, or vibrator.

The cream, available by prescription, comes in dosages from 0.01 mg to 1.5 mg, and should not be used right before intercourse, since activity will cause it to leak out. Over time, the cream may make such an improvement in vaginal tissue elasticity and stability that you can decrease the dosage (some women use it only once every three weeks after they've been on it for a few months). Your doctor will advise you not to use this cream more frequently than twice weekly, since if you do so, estrogen will be absorbed into the bloodstream and may be associated with risks of other estrogen products (see Chapter 7 for details on dosage and administration).

You can also try the over-the-counter progesterone cream derived from wild yam root (available in many health food stores). This cream will alleviate burning and itching, and may provide the same relief as estrogen cream for some women.

Q: Will HRT help me to have an orgasm?
Probably not. However, it may help out with other problems that keep you from relaxing and letting go. If you were previously orgasmic but are no more, HRT may make a big difference, particularly when boosted with the

hormone testosterone. (See Chapter 7 for a discussion of combining estrogen and testosterone to improve libido.) Amplifying your hormonal output should restore desire and function to your sexuality.

Q: Are there any herbs that will make me feel sexier?
Herbal remedies that will restore thickness and moisture to the vagina include tincture of motherwort or chaste tree (Vitex). In order to keep vaginal tissues strong and elastic, try a sitz bath of comfrey root five to ten minutes three or four times a week. Chewing dong quai root (available in Chinese markets) is said to increase vaginal lubrication.

Questions About Incontinence

The deep, dark secret of midlife and older life is that many women cannot retain their urine and are too embarrassed to ask their physicians for help. This humiliating problem is in many cases due to a loss of estrogen, and it can often be rectified by both replacement hormones, special exercises, and a variety of behavioral strategies.

Q: What is incontinence?
Incontinence is the inability to control urinary output.

Q: Is urinary incontinence common?
Extremely so. About 20 to 30 percent of all women have some form of incontinence, and the statistic rises to 38 percent in women over sixty. The probability of becoming incontinent increases with age and tends to be more prevalent in those who are overweight or have borne many children, and in women who have had hysterectomies.

Q: What is the cause?

There are usually several causes. Natural changes in bladder function occur with aging and with a decrease in the gonadal hormones estrogen and progesterone.

The urethra (the tube leading from the bladder to the urethral opening where we pass urine) loses mucosal cells, which contain estrogen receptors, after menopause. Without sufficient estrogen, the urethra also doesn't get as much blood vessel engorgement in the lower urinary tract as it used to. The number of cells and the blood vessel engorgement are both important in helping to sustain sufficient pressure so that the urethra closes entirely after voiding. Less estrogen means less pressure to close the urethra.

Pelvic floor muscles also become less elastic as estrogen supplies decrease. This means that any sudden increase in pressure in the abdomen (like coughing or sneezing) stresses the bladder, making it difficult to retain urine.

There may be other health factors involved—urinary tract infections and urethral thinning due to a rapid decline in estrogen are the most common—but incontinence can also be caused by fibroid tumors in the uterus that irritate the bladder and cause so much pressure, you can't hold your urine.

Q: Is it important for me to tell my doctor about my incontinence? Can't I just handle this myself?

The faster you get help, the better, because treating the condition in its early stages is much more successful than treating it when it's more advanced.

Some women are too embarrassed to say anything about incontinence and feel they are destined to a life in adult diapers. This is completely untrue!

Perhaps the worst part of this condition is the humiliation factor; a woman in midlife may simply try to deny what's happening and use a "Band-Aid" remedy such as incontinence pads. But because there are so many excellent programs and remedies, it's important to get treatment.

Don't keep quiet about it. Talk to your doctor and you will find a sympathetic ear and strategies to help remedy the situation.

Q: Are there several types of incontinence?

Yes. You may suffer from *stress* incontinence or *urge* incontinence.

With stress incontinence, you may pass a small amount of urine when you cough, sneeze, laugh, or while doing some physical activity that takes effort. Stress incontinence is quite common at this time of life, since urethral thinning and loss of muscle tone make pressure from the uterus on the bladder and pelvic floor muscles difficult to manage. Additionally, in smokers, the problem can be exacerbated by coughing, which puts pressure on the abdomen, which in turn presses down on the bladder.

If you examine a model of the female reproductive system, you will see that the bladder lies directly beside the uterus. Sometimes the contractions that take place in the uterus when you are sexually stimulated can cause the bladder to leak some of its contents.

Urge incontinence (being unable to wait to go to the bathroom, even if you've just gone, or wetting the bed at night) is also common, and it may have structural and behavioral components. The physical cause is an inability to control the detrusor muscle, which usually contracts to hold back urine, but no longer functions properly due to loss of elasticity and slowing signals from the muscle to the nerve endings in the brain. Other causes of urge incontinence may be infection, inflammation, bladder stones, or stool impaction.

Mixed incontinence occurs when both syndromes occur together. Sometimes the problem is a "dropped bladder," which makes emptying too easy. Occasionally women who have borne many children have a predisposition to urethral and pelvic floor weakness.

Q: What are some risk factors for incontinence?

It has been found that heavy or obese women, those who have been hysterectomized, and those who are in their seventies and eighties are at greater risk. In younger women, the number of children seems to have an effect on continence—those who have no children are at the least risk. Several diseases also seem to put you at greater risk, such as stroke, chronic obstructive pulmonary disease, and diabetes. Women who are in overall poor general health are also more at risk for incontinence.

Q: Is cigarette smoking in any way connected with incontinence?

Yes. People who smoke tend to cough a great deal, and this is one trigger for stress incontinence. Nicotine also has adverse effects on nearly every tissue in the body— including the kidneys and bladder. Stopping smoking could not only save your life but also keep you continent.

Q: I get up to go to the bathroom a couple of times a night. Does this mean I'm incontinent?

No. Many women who are used to voiding every few hours during the day repeat this pattern at night. You may wish to try restricting your liquids after six P.M.— although that doesn't help some women and may lead to constipation—but it's far better to drink more and urinate more than to not drink enough. Most urologists recommend that flushing your kidneys with eight to ten glasses of water a day and going to the bathroom more often may help to prevent urinary tract infections.

Q: Every once in a while, I leak a little urine when I have an orgasm. Is that normal, and what can I do to prevent it?

This is one symptom of stress incontinence, but no, it is not to be expected. You should void your bladder completely before any sexual activity, and you may wish to put a towel under you.

You might be interested to know that some women have the ability to "female ejaculate"—they pass a clear, odorless liquid when they climax that is produced near the G-spot at the front of the anterior wall of the vagina. You'll be able to tell the difference by whether there's an odor of urine or not. So it's conceivable that you're not incontinent, just very sexy.

Q: What tests would my doctor do to find the cause of my incontinence?

S/he would take a thorough medical history, asking about any problems with urination, how many times you get up during the night or whether you wet the bed, whether you have trouble beginning to void, frequent urinary tract infections, or painful urination. S/he would also want to know how much coffee, cola, and alcohol you consume daily (these are all urinary tract irritants), and what medications you take. Chronic use of diuretics for weight loss is a typical cause of urinary tract dysfunction.

Then your doctor would ask you to give a clean catch urine sample, which s/he would examine for sugar and protein. S/he would do a urine culture to see if any infection was present. S/he would also do a complete pelvic and bimanual exam with a Pap smear and would examine your vagina, vulva, and labia.

S/he would also ask you to keep a diary that designated the times of voiding and amount of fluids you drank that day.

If natural methods of controlling urine function (see

below) were making no difference, s/he would probably go on to order an X ray or ultrasound test; possibly, a cystoscopy to look inside the bladder; a bladder-filling cystometrogram to record the pressure in the bladder at varying stages of filling; and other tests of bladder function (urodynamics).

Q: Will HRT or other medications help with leakage or incontinence?

HRT might help with urge incontinence, though probably not with stress incontinence. Estrogen cream used two or three times weekly at bedtime may restore good tone to the area and give better control of the detrusor muscle. It seems to be most effective in combination with other, natural therapies.

The most commonly used drugs are anticholinergic drugs such as oxybutynin for urge incontinence, and alpha-agonists such as phenylpropanolamine and ephedrine. These drugs can relax the bladder, increasing capacity and also increasing urethral resistance. Another commonly used drug is imipramine, an antidepressant that also helps to inhibit the bladder muscle.

Estrogen cream and other medications are usually used in combination with biofeedback, Kegel exercises, and vaginal cones (see below).

Q: Are there natural techniques that will help to control my bladder?

There are many—you just have to be dedicated to using them. Everything from Kegel exercises to biofeedback, to devices that you hold inside the vagina, to herbs and homeopathic remedies will help your incontinence. All of these can be used alone or in combination with medication.

Q: Whenever I finish urinating, I feel like I have to go again. What should I do about this?

It's very important to empty your bladder completely every time—pressing down on the pubic bone while you're urinating will help to clear everything out.

Q: What are Kegels and how do they help?

The Kegel (named for the doctor who counseled his postpartum patients to use it) is a squeeze of the pubococcygeal muscles (those between the vagina and the anus). In order to do one Kegel, you imagine that you are urinating and then you shut off the flow of urine. This opens and closes the muscles around the entrance to the vagina and keeps them elastic. It also tones the urethra (preventing the leakage of urine during sexual activity). Kegels will strengthen pelvic floor muscles and help to control your bladder.

You can practice Kegels at any time (no one will know!), doing six sets of ten Kegels three times a day. When you get better at them, you can speed up the pace and also try to alternate squeezing the front muscles (around the vagina) and the back muscles (around the anus).

Q: Are there herbs and homeopathic remedies that can help?

A daily cup of dried teasel root (1 tablespoon to 1 cup of water boiled for about ten minutes) will strengthen the bladder.

Antispasmodic herbs will help with urge incontinence. Try 10 to 20 drops of black cohosh tincture once or twice a day for several weeks or as needed. You can also use teas of ginger, catnip, or corn silk at any time.

Homeopathic remedies you might try include pulsatilla and zincum met.

Q: Does what I eat and drink affect my urinary control?

Yes, it certainly does. Eliminate or reduce coffee (caffeinated and decaffeinated), alcohol, carbonated beverages, aspartame (Nutrasweet), and refined sugar—these can all aggravate a hyperactive bladder. You may also wish to cut down on very cold foods, hot and spicy foods and seasonings, citrus fruits, tomatoes, and pineapple, which are all bladder irritants.

Q: Are there behavioral methods that might help me?

There are excellent behavioral programs where you strictly schedule your toileting and drinking. Try to measure out what you drink so that you consume equal amounts throughout the day. You will have to arrange your day so that you can void your bladder every hour while you're awake. For some women, an hour can seem an eternity, but it's best to try for that regularity when you're first learning bladder control. In order to get results from this training, you have to stick to this schedule, even if it means wetting a pad. After three or four successful days, increase your time by fifteen to thirty minutes. Every seven to ten days, increase the time again.

Q: I've heard biofeedback is effective. How does it work?

Biofeedback is successful for one-half to two-thirds of the women who try it. An electromyography (EMG) machine is used to record the amount of pressure the pelvic muscles can exert and the results are depicted on a screen. As you get better at contracting these muscles, you can see incremental changes in your data on the screen. You can go to a clinic to learn to use these machines or purchase your own.

Q: Is it true that you can use electrical stimulation to control the bladder? Does this hurt?

Yes, you can, and there is no pain involved. Functional electrical stimulation is used as a treatment for urge and stress incontinence. This is similar to the type of pain relief available in a TENS (transcutaneous electrical nerve stimulation) unit, a small device that is applied to the skin and puts out impulses that block pain responses. For bladder control, a vaginal or rectal probe is inserted to give a mild, painless stimulus that makes the muscles contract. You can adjust the frequency and intensity of the electrical current according to your comfort level.

Q: What are vaginal cones, and how do you use them?

Weighted vaginal cones can strengthen the pubococcygeal area. These small weights (shaped something like fishing buoys) are placed at the entrance to the vaginal barrel. You have to squeeze around them to keep them from falling out. You wear them twice a day for fifteen minutes at a time, walking around and doing light exercise. As you train your muscles, you progress to heavier cones. (See the Resource Guide, page 224, if you wish to order these cones.)

Q: Is it true that if you wear a tampon, you can control your urine?

Some doctors recommend mechanical devices to help with bladder control. A tampon, diaphragm, or pessary (a rubber device placed inside the vagina that supports the uterus) can help to retain muscular support in the pubococcygeal area.

Q: What is the Introl Bladder Neck Support Prosthesis (BNSP)?

This device, developed by an Australian gynecologist, supports the neck of the bladder with a flexible silicone ring that has two prongs at one end. The support is inserted in the vagina and sits on the pelvic floor, pushing up on the neck of the bladder.

The BNSP has been found 80 percent effective for stress incontinence in women who were tested with the device over a three-year period. Some women leave it in place all day; others just put it in before exercise or sexual activity.

Q: If I've tried everything else and nothing works, will I have to have surgery?

Possibly. Since surgery is really a last resort (and isn't always successful), your physician might try injections of collagen into the neck of the bladder. This increases bulk in the wall of the urethra, which allows for tighter closure.

Surgery is usually only recommended for women with severe stress incontinence, bladder tumors, or severe prolapse of the bladder, vagina, or rectum.

Questions About Alzheimer's Disease

The disease that ravages the mind and eventually destroys bodily function strikes fear in the hearts of many women who have been told that they may "go crazy" at menopause. Of course, this is an untrue, unfair stereotype—misplacing things and forgetting words are menopausal complaints that pass and have nothing to do with senile dementia.

It is true, however, that more women develop Alzheimer's than men, and it generally begins in midlife. Preliminary findings are very sketchy, but there is hope that this disease, caused by a dramatic loss of brain cells, may respond, at least partially, to replacement estrogen.

Q: What is Alzheimer's disease?

Alzheimer's (named after Alois Alzheimer, a German

pathologist who identified this syndrome sometime after the turn of the century) is the most common type of senile dementia, a nervous system disease.

Q: How many individuals get Alzheimer's?
Roughly two to three million Americans a year and approximately 50 percent of all women over 85 contract this disease. Because it has so many complications, it ranks among the top ten causes of death in this country.

Q: Why does it occur?
Although aging in general causes a loss of neurons in the brain, the dramatic loss in cells present in Alzheimer's is abnormal. This disease is also characterized by plaques and tangles that develop on and among the neurons. Current research indicates that a genetic component (similar to that in Down's syndrome) may partly account for the development of this disease. Other factors that come into play are the lack of the neurotransmitter acetylcholine, cytotoxic (cell poisoning) immune factors, aluminum deposition in the brain cells, some viruses, and lesions in particular areas of the brain.

Q: My mother had Alzheimer's. Does this mean I will get it, too?
It's not a given that you will inherit it. There are currently tests to genotype you for the apolipoprotein E, which appears in 40 percent of all Alzheimer's cases. However, just because you test positive for the apolipoprotein doesn't mean you will necessarily get the disease, and even if you don't have the gene, you may still get the disease. It does mean, however, that you can consider yourself at risk. If you are the type of person who feels she must plan for the future in great detail or get early treatment when it is available, you may wish to be tested.

Q: What's the typical age that a person might contract Alzheimer's?

Although there are those under the age of sixty who begin to show signs of the disease, it is far more common in the elderly. After age sixty-five, the prevalence of all types of dementia doubles every four to five years and is greater in women than in men.

Q: If I constantly forget things, does this mean I'm getting Alzheimer's?

No! Memory loss (particularly short-term memory, such as phone numbers or where you parked the car at the mall) is a perfectly normal consequence of menopausal change. Although the old stereotype of "Mom's in menopause and she's going crazy" is unfortunately still around and may relate to occasional lapses of memory, there is no reason to be concerned about normal forgetfulness.

Q: Will HRT help me to remember things?

Many women find that HRT assists in routine memory loss, possibly because estrogen does increase blood flow to the brain. There's also the placebo factor—women tend to feel more confident and therefore don't have so many anxious moments where they lose their train of thought. Another factor is that hormonal supplementation enhances the plasticity of neurons, thereby making the nervous system function more effectively. But other ways to remember things are writing things down, keeping a bulletin board in your home and office, and playing mental games to keep brain cells active. In one game, "I Packed My Suitcase," you place imaginary items in a suitcase and challenge yourself to repeat them in order.

Q: Suppose it's not just forgetfulness. What are actual symptoms of Alzheimer's?

The diagnosis of Alzheimer's is not made until the

following symptoms have been gradually progressing for at least six months. The condition is judged by:

- impairment of at least two cognitive abilities (attention, learning, memory, or orientation) *and*
- impairment of one symbolic skill-calculation, abstraction, or comprehension *and*
- problems in at least one life area, such as work, family, peer relationships, or social functioning

Q: How is Alzheimer's typically treated?

Some studies have shown that the problem may be a lack of a particular neurotransmitter, or brain hormone. Some researchers advocate giving increased amounts of acetylcholine to patients, though not much progress has been made in this direction.

HRT, if started right after menopause, has been shown in some small studies to be preventive against Alzheimer's; however, a great deal more investigation has to be done on the relation of hormones to this disease before it can be prescribed routinely for this purpose.

Q: Why would replacement estrogen help in the treatment of Alzheimer's?

Estrogen may promote the growth of certain types of nerve cells that can help to improve memory function. Researchers are currently hopeful that estrogen therapy can prevent the death and disappearance of nerve cells, a process characterized by Alzheimer's disease.

Q: What has ERT been able to do for Alzheimer's patients?

Early research is promising. In several studies from two Massachusetts clinics, it was found that women who had used replacement estrogen were less likely to develop Alzheimer's. In several Japanese studies, it was found that replacing estrogen in those who had already been diagnosed made significant improvements in social skills and ability to function.

Currently, the first large-scale study of Alzheimer's prevention in healthy older women is under way at the Bowman Gray School of Medicine in Winston-Salem, North Carolina. The researchers will be trying to discover whether a specific subcomponent of Premarin, the hormone equilin, may protect and stimulate brain neurons without posing the threat of breast or uterine cancer. Studies in laboratory animals with equilin have given new hope to Alzheimer's researchers. The Women's Health Initiative Memory Study (WHI-MS) should have more answers when their results are tabulated in 2006.

One American study found that the addition of a progestin had unfavorable results—which would mean that hysterectomized women with Alzheimer's would be the most likely candidates for this therapy. Other studies confirm the findings that progestin reverses the action of estrogen on blood flow in the brain and therefore can be detrimental in the treatment of Alzheimer's.

Questions About Depression

Nearly every woman has the "blues" sometimes. Clinical depression, on the other hand, is a severe and debilitating condition that can be treated. Although antidepressant medications are usually the first line of treatment for depression, estrogen appears to be very beneficial for some women who are diagnosed with this condition.

Q: Does every woman get depressed when she goes through menopause?
Absolutely not. Although this time of life—like puberty and childbirth—is rife with emotional upheaval, it is not a

given that every woman falls apart at midlife. It is far more common to be depressed at midlife if you have suffered depressions earlier in life. In several studies, only 25 percent of women felt slightly depressed at menopause.

Q: I go through times of the week or month when I feel really blue. Am I depressed?

You may be, but it's more probable that you are at a downswing of your personal emotional cycle, which is common in many women. If you happen to be under a lot of stress, or ill, or have a family member out of work or needing to be cared for, it's likely that some days you might not be as successful coping with problems as others.

Q: What are my risk factors for depression?

If you're female, you are twice as likely to become depressed as your male friends and relatives, and this statistic is as true for female adolescents as it is for those in their fifties. If you are going through a major life change—divorce, death of a loved one, end or beginning of a career, moving across the country, etc.—these additional stresses would add to the likelihood of your feeling overwhelmed.

Q: What is the definition of clinical depression?

Depression is a mental, emotional, physical, and spiritual state that distorts your impressions of events and people. On the one hand, you may feel hopeless and sad most of the time if you're depressed, or you may feel angry and put upon; on the other hand, you may swear that nothing is wrong. Some depressions manifest themselves in emotional despair, while others are masked in physical symptoms similar to those we get when very stressed out—stomachaches, headaches, palpitations, and dizziness may all be signs of depression.

Approximately 15 million Americans feel depressed each year, although only 1.5 million seek treatment. The majority of depressions clear up by themselves within six to nine months with or without treatment. Time heals.

It's important to diagnose depression accurately. The following are changes that you may notice if you are feeling depressed:

- lack of interest in activities and people
- sadness and pessimism about everything
- inability to enjoy yourself
- irritability
- difficulty concentrating
- changes in appetite, weight, and sleep patterns
- loss of libido
- indecisiveness

If the depression continues and worsens, the following symptoms may appear:

- lack of self-esteem, feeling unworthy
- exhaustion
- abandoning work and home responsibilities
- abandoning personal hygiene
- inability to communicate with others
- feelings of impending doom, utter hopelessness
- thoughts of death

If you experience four or more of the above symptoms and they last for two weeks or longer, you may be in a depression and should seek professional advice immediately.

Q: Where does depression come from?

There is a great deal of interesting speculation about the genetic causes of depression, but experts are as yet uncertain as to the hereditary components of this illness. We do know there are physiological, psychological, and social causes:

Physiological causes: Certain brain neurotransmitters may not be secreted in sufficient amounts to alleviate mood disorders. The chemicals *serotonin, melatonin,* and *dopamine* are the most important to our sense of well-being. When the nerves are robbed of these neurotransmitters, they can't send messages to other nerves, and depression results. (The opposite problem, having excess neurotransmitter production, can cause hyperactivity and a manic state.)

Psychological causes: Our personalities greatly determine who we are and what we will make of the raw ingredients bequeathed to us through our DNA. A resilient individual who is abused in childhood may still grow up unscathed by depression, whereas a chronic worrier or dependent person may feel overwhelmed by the smallest incidents. If you think you deserve to feel miserable, chances are you will learn to feel that way.

Social causes: Being abused, poor, neglected, or separated from loved ones can encourage an incipient depression. It has been found, for example, that older women whose spouses have died and whose family has moved away often develop what is known as a "failure to thrive." When no one needs you, you feel unwanted and depressed—which can in turn exacerbate physical symptoms that can lead to illness or death.

Circumstantial causes: If you have undergone a mastectomy or hysterectomy, it is understandable that you might feel negative and robbed of your femininity. If you were mugged or raped, you may feel as though you can't cope with the guilt and anguish of the experience. These can all lead to depression.

Q: If I feel depressed, isn't it just because of my depressing symptoms such as hot flashes and vaginal dryness?

Not necessarily, since those symptoms don't depress all

women. However, several studies have shown that the peak of troublesome psychological symptoms coincides with the biggest decline in natural estrogens—which typically takes place a few years *before* menopause.

If, however, you are suffering from night sweats and haven't slept properly in weeks, this can certainly make you feel depressed and miserable. So can other problems such as headaches, joint pains, and palpitations, or not taking care of yourself by eating and exercising well, thereby becoming less resistant to disease.

Q: What type of doctor should I see for depression?

If you currently see a family practice physician, gynecologist, or endocrinologist, s/he is the first one you should consult about these problems. S/he may wish to refer you for short-term counseling to a psychologist, clinical social worker, or marital counselor, depending on the problem. S/he may also suggest that you consider hormone replacement therapy first, to see whether there is a hormonal component to your depression.

If three or four months of HRT does not make a difference, s/he may suggest that you consult a psychiatrist so that your problems can be handled both with talk therapy and drug therapy. Although really serious depressions do respond well to various drugs, *no* drug will be effective on a long-term basis unless you are discussing the roots of the problem in therapy at the same time.

Q: Does HRT help to alleviate depression?

One part of it does; the other doesn't. Estrogen helps to modulate the production of serotonin in the brain—the neurotransmitter that gives us a sense of well-being (and which is the major component of Prozac, Zoloft, and other popular "feel-good" drugs). So the estrogen portion of your regimen lifts the spirits.

But the progesterone portion seems to bring a lot of

women down. This hormone, which is released during the second half of the female cycle, has been implicated in creating unpleasant PMS-type symptoms such as irritability, fatigue, and the blues. When estrogen levels are elevated with HRT or ERT throughout your cycle, they can often counteract these symptoms.

Q: Would I take a normal low dose of oral estrogen for depression?

The Estraderm patch has been used most frequently in the treatment of depression, and the dosage is usually 0.1 mg, changed twice weekly. Slightly higher daily oral doses (1.25 mg) seem to be more effective than the standard oral dose of 0.625 mg. You must also use a progestin if you still have a uterus. (See Chapter 7 for a full discussion of prescriptions and dosages.)

Q: Are there other drugs I can use for depression?

If you see a general practice physician or a psychotherapist instead of an endocrinologist for your symptoms, you may be prescribed one of the many antidepressants or mood-elevating drugs that are on the market. Probably hundreds of thousands of women who have visited doctors at the "change of life" over the decades have been told that it's natural to feel down and blue, and consequently that the only course of action is to take what used to be called "nerve pills." From Lydia Pinkham's Tonic at the turn of the century to Miltown in the 1950s to Valium (a depressant that brings you down rather than up!) in the 1980s to today's high-tech family of selective serotonin reuptake inhibitors (SSRIs) like Prozac, Paxil, Effexor, Serzone, and Zoloft, there has long been a pharmaceutical answer for depression.

It may be that HRT alone will not be sufficient to lift a serious depression and that medication combined with psychotherapy may help you through a difficult spell. It's worth noting that many doctors still prescribe tranquil-izers (Valium, Xanax, Ativan) to patients who really need antidepressants (Elavil, Prozac, Effexor, and others). You should question your physician carefully when discussing which drug s/he feels you should take.

Another possibility is that you have a condition where you feel manic for a cycle and then depressed for a cycle. You may have bipolar disorder and require a drug such as Wellbutrin to control your condition. However, it is essen-tial that you have a clear diagnosis before any attempt is made to medicate the symptoms.

Remember, however, that all psychopharmaceutical drugs have side effects, and you should be wary of taking them when you are already at a time in life when minor physical changes—from headache to gastrointestinal dis-orders to joint pains—may appear without any additional chemical stimuli.

Q: What are some natural treatments I can use for depression?

There are literally dozens of treatments that have been shown to be very successful:

Exercise: If you currently do no physical activity, this is the most important change you can make. Get out every day and walk, swim, bike, jog, dance, or play racket sports. This stimulates the production of beta endorphins—those feel-good chemicals in your brain that act as natural opi-ates to alleviate pain (mental or physical). Exercise also gives you a firmer, more fit body—which in itself imparts a great sense of pride and self-confidence.

Nutrition: What you eat can certainly make a difference in your mental health—get rid of junk food, refined sugar, caffeine, and red meat and see how much better you feel. Consume small meals more frequently, and make sure they are high in complex carbohydrates, fresh fruits, and vegetables. You should also include lots of estrogenic foods such as tofu, tempeh, miso, and Mexican yams.

Vitamin and mineral supplementation: All the B vitamins, particularly B_1, B_6, and B_{12}, are known as the stress vitamins and can assist your body in managing stress on a daily basis. Tryptophan, the amino acid that is the precursor to serotonin, often declines in depressed people. You can get this amino acid in warmed milk, bananas, kiwi, and other foods, and it is available (usually in combination with other herbs or amino acids) as a sleeping remedy in health food stores.

Herbs: Saint-John's-wort, which restores the nervous system, has been found to be enormously effective in the treatment of depression. Ginkgo biloba is renowned for its ability to help with memory loss and has been used clinically to slow the progression of Alzheimer's. Excellent herbs for anxiety are kava-kava and valerian. The latter is also good for insomnia.

Other herbs that are useful for treating depression are balm, black hellebore, borage, clove, fo-ti, gingseng, rosemary, sage, or thyme.

Homeopathy: You may wish to try the following remedies: Arsenicum album, pulsatilla, ignatia, or sepia.

Acupressure: You may press on the following points: GB20 (between the neck muscles at the base of the skull), UB38 (half an inch out from the muscles bordering the spine beside the top of the shoulder blade), the third eye point (between your brows), UB23 and UB47 (two inches and four inches out from the spine at waist level), and ST13 (just below the collarbone on both sides near the shoulders).

Face and scalp massage: Rub your hands together until you feel the warmth between them, then cup them over your eyes. From here, move down to your cheeks and press the tops of your cheekbones below your eyes. Next, massage underneath each cheekbone, starting close to the nose and working your way out to the ears. Move your hands to the back of your head, placing your thumbs on the base of your skull and your fingertips on top of your head. Slowly work your thumbs up the back of your head. Place all your fingers and thumbs on your scalp and massage the skin, under the hair. Breathe deeply as you do this exercise.

Meditation and breathing: Allow yourself a quiet twenty minutes a day to sit with the phone turned off and nowhere to go. Now just concentrate on inhaling and exhaling, clearing your mind of everything else. By physically calming your body with breath, you will start the process of calming yourself mentally as well.

Prayer: Many women find that giving themselves over to the authority of a higher power can be a great release from their daily burdens. Whether you believe in a deity or not, prayer allows you to connect up with the life force of the universe, which is bigger and stronger than any depression.

Self-esteem enhancement: Give yourself a sense of control in your life. Women who feel they are accomplishing something, who can make a difference in their personal and professional lives, tend to be able to manage stress much better. If you have a job where you make decisions for yourself and others, you are less likely to feel helpless and victimized. However, women who tend to feel that they are dependent on "the system" or a partner, who are run ragged with caregiving duties for children or elderly parents, or who feel that no one pays attention to their concerns are those at highest risk for depression (and other serious illnesses such as cancer and cardiovascular disorders).

Chapter Ten

Finding Natural Ways to Replace Estrogen

Suppose you cannot take hormone replacement therapy because you've had an estrogen-dependent cancer or have a strong family history of cancer. Or perhaps you're just leery of taking medication when you're not sick. You have no risk factors for heart disease or osteoporosis, but you are more fatigued than you used to be, and you'd like to be able to add more energy and vitality to your life. Is there some way to do this *without* a prescription for hormones?

Happily, there is a way to replenish some of the hormones you're losing that is completely natural. You can make changes in your eating, your exercising, and your supplementation so as to alleviate many of the signs and signals of menopause.

All About Phytosterols

Plants produce estrogenic substances that can be used by animals and humans. Although they aren't exactly like the estradiol, estrone, and estriol that the body produces, eating these plants can be beneficial as part of a natural program to alleviate menopausal complaints and perhaps to retard bone loss and offer protection to the heart as well.

Q: What is a dietary phytosterol?

This is a particular class of compounds found in the diet with a molecular structure similar to estrogen. When ingested, phytosterols bind to estrogen helpers and have estrogenlike effects in the body, bumping up the effectiveness of the body's own estrogen. As you eat more of these plant compounds, your body is better able to manufacture its own hormones, or keep its level of hormones on an even keel.

Q: What are some sources of dietary phytosterols?

The most common sources are soybeans and flaxseed (which can be taken as an oil). At least three hundred herbs also contain these compounds. (See below for the most common estrogenic herbs that can be taken as teas, infusions, or tinctures.)

Q: Is there scientific proof that phytosterols can reduce heart disease and osteoporosis?

No. As yet, scientists don't feel that dietary estrogens can be used to prevent disease. However, in premenopausal women, a high-soy diet was found to prolong the menstrual cycle and, more specifically, to lengthen the first half of the cycle prior to ovulation when estrogen is the predominant hormone. It also reduced the mid-cycle surge of hormones that typically causes PMS-like problems.

Soy Products That Help to Protect Your Heart and Reduce Menopausal Symptoms

One of the best and easiest ways to revamp your nutritional program is to add ingredients derived from the soybean. The estrogenic qualities of this plant help the body to use its own estrogen more effectively.

Q: Why are soy products good sources of natural estrogens?

Soy products contain chemicals that defend the plant against disease or environmental hazards like radiation and drought. These chemicals, called *phytoalexins*, are common to many plants. However, one form of the phytoalexins, *isoflavones*, is unique to soy and chickpeas (garbanzos). In the human body, isoflavones are converted by intestinal bacteria into *phytosterols*, or estrogen look-alike molecules. They have an estrogenic effect on the body when ingested. (Men can eat soy products without fear of overfeminization, since the testosterone they produce is more than enough to compensate for dietary estrogenic effects.)

Many of the "natural" progesterone and estrogen products sold by pharmacies (see the Resource Guide, pages 224–226) are derived from soybean plants.

Q: How do we know that soy is beneficial to menopausal women?

There is no word in Japanese for "hot flash," and very few women over the age of fifty who eat a traditional Japanese diet ever develop heart disease or breast cancer. One of the staples of this diet is soy—the foods made from this bean are tofu, tempeh, miso, and soy protein powder.

Nutrition is a big influence on our body's changing chemistry. A report in the *New England Journal of Medicine* in August 1995 confirms this fact. The authors of the

study found that soy protein significantly lowered cholesterol in participants who were at high risk for heart disease because of their elevated cholesterol. The higher
their risk, the more their levels dropped after eating soy.
If their total cholesterol was way up at 300 and their LDLs
were a big percentage of that, they could cut their cholesterol by 20 percent in just one month.

Q: What does soy do to protect the heart?

The phytosterols in soy change LDL molecules so that
they can't adhere to artery walls. This means that although soy consumption can't prevent a heart attack or
any other cardiovascular event, it reduces your likelihood
of *developing* heart disease. Soybeans also contain two
amino acids, lysine and argenine, which lower insulin
levels, causing the liver to produce less cholesterol.

**Q: How long would it take me to reduce my risk of
heart disease by eating soy?**

A six-month program of a diet high in soy will give you
a 10 to 15 percent reduction in blood cholesterol, and
this amounts to a 20 to 30 percent reduction in heart disease risk.

Q: Will eating soy lower my risk of breast cancer?

It might, but only if you are a dedicated soy eater
throughout your reproductive years. During the first half
of a typical menstrual cycle, breast tissue is not active.
There's no new cell growth until just before ovulation,
when we get a surge of estradiol (the strongest form of
human estrogen). The estradiol binds with estrogen
receptors to start up new cell growth, which causes the
commonly tender breasts we get prior to a period.

But if you consume a great deal of soy in your diet,
you can avoid this problem. One of the phytosterols
in soy, *genistein*, is a particularly influential chemical.

Even though this plant chemical is only about one one-hundredth as strong as estradiol, it can lock onto estrogen receptors in the breast and block the activity of estradiol. This will prolong the first half of your cycle and stem the midcycle hormonal surge.

Over many years of eating soy, if you can prolong your cycle from twenty-eight to thirty-two days, you thereby cut down on the number of times breast tissue is stimulated. It has been shown that there is less incidence of breast cancer in cultures where women bear many children and nurse them for years (thereby having fewer periods).

Q: Is it too late for me to change my diet if I'm no longer menstruating?

If you are in perimenopause, or even if you are post-menopausal, you may still be able to block the development of a tumor or slow its progress by changing your dietary habits. Breast cancer is a very slow-growing cancer—there can be a delay of ten to thirty years from the appearance of the first cancer cell to its detection as a lump. This means that if you have a family history or are at high risk for breast cancer, it makes a great deal of sense to start eating a high-soy diet (at least 50 grams daily).

Q: What will eating soy do to lower my risk of osteoporosis?

Just as genistein is important in the breast cancer picture, so another phytosterol, *ipriflavone*, may be a contender in the battle against osteoporosis. In a study on postmenopausal women with low bone mass, it was found that taking 600 to 1,200 mg of ipriflavone daily for a year resulted in a significant increase in the bone mineral density of the radius of the arm. The therapy is currently approved for treatment of osteoporosis in Japan, Italy, and Hungary.

In America, this is still an experimental therapy, but as more studies confirm the findings, soy consumption may be deemed one method of preventing or treating osteoporosis.

Q: Will soy products help other menopausal problems?

Most women find great relief from a variety of menopausal symptoms in a high-soy diet. Remember that phytosterols do not work like a magic bullet, zinging toward one target organ and "fixing" what's wrong. Rather, they work in a holistic fashion on the whole body. The estrogenic elements in plants nourish the ovaries, adrenals, and the pituitary gland in the brain. You can use diet effectively to change the biochemical environment of your body.

Many menopausal symptoms appear to be caused by a radical fluctuation in hormonal output rather than simply a deficiency. But phytoestrogens can block the action of human estrogens, thus stemming the big swings in output. Because of the estrogenic effects of these chemicals, a diet high in phytosterols can alleviate or reduce the intensity and frequency of hot flashes; it can reduce the flow of perimenopausal bleeding; and there is anecdotal evidence that it can work on other complaints such as sleep disturbances and emotional imbalance.

Q: How much soy should I eat to replenish the hormones I'm lacking?

The *New England Journal* study indicates that we need a lot of soy to make a difference in our cholesterol. The benefits start to kick in when you're eating at least 25 grams of soy daily, but twice that amount is recommended if you have very high cholesterol to start with. A soy burger contains about 18 grams; a glass of soy milk about 8 grams; a cake of tofu has about 16 grams.

If you have very high cholesterol (and women's levels do elevate at menopause), you should double the amount of soy you're eating. A diet of 47 grams of soy protein daily (about two soy burgers and an eight-ounce glass of soy milk) will cut cholesterol levels by 9.3 percent in a month, unless your cholesterol level is very high to begin with.

Q: This is a huge amount! What else would I be able to eat?

The good thing about this diet is that you'll be too filled with beneficial nutrients to fit in much animal protein. The reduction in red meat and dairy will also lower your cholesterol.

You should plan your meals to include fresh vegetables, fruits, and whole grains in addition to the soy. Drink lots of water and herbal teas as well.

Q: What are some of the foods I can eat that are made of soy?

Start with the soybeans themselves—you can buy the dried beans in your supermarket or health food store. Soak them first (several hours or overnight) and then cook. They can be used in a variety of dishes, from soups to casseroles. You can also get them canned—it's usually best to drain them before using. You can buy fresh soybeans in Asian markets and add them to stir-fry dishes, or they can also be sprouted to add to a salad. Soynuts are sold as snacks and are much better for you than potato chips!

You can purchase "burgers," or TVP (texturized vegetable protein), which are made from defatted soy flour that has been compressed into a patty shape (you can also make your own from a mix); there are also "No-Dogs" and soy sausages available in most supermarkets or health food stores.

Tofu, or bean curd, is a cake of curdled soy milk. The different textures—soft, medium, and firm—offer a wide range of uses. You can chop it and add it to a stir-fry with vegetables and noodles, use it to replace some meat in a meatloaf or casserole, or you can substitute it for an egg when you're baking and even make mayonnaise with it. There are also soy cheeses and frozen desserts available in your supermarket or health food store.

Tempeh and miso may be the best soy products to use, because they are made from the whole soybean. Tempeh is a combination of soybeans and grains and makes a tasty burger; miso is a salty fermented soy paste that can be used in soups and sauces. These products are available in Asian markets and health food stores.

Soy protein powder is found in health food stores—you can add this to sauces, or sprinkle it into vegetable dishes to thicken them a bit. You can also use it as filler in a vegetarian "meatloaf" mix using ground nuts, squash, onions, and cooked rice. You can also mix it in fruit juice or make a shake with it.

Soy oil is about 50 percent linolenic acid, the essential ingredient in evening primrose oil and borage oil. It is also used to produce vitamin E supplements. (See Chapter 3 for a description of the advantages of these oils for menopausal women.)

Estrogen-Rich Herbal Supplements for Menopause

Instead of just eating your hormones, you can supplement with herbs taken as infusions or tinctures. The phytosterols are generally found in perennial roots, leaf buds, and hard berries.

Q: Which herbs are rich in phytosterols?

There are about three hundred of them, but the ones most commonly recommended for menopause are burdock root, licorice root, dong quai, wild yam root (*Dioscorea*), and motherwort. These are sometimes taken separately, and sometimes brewed together. Other herbs that are beneficial at the time of menopause are ginseng (which is highly estrogenic), false unicorn, anise, sage, black cohosh, and raspberry leaf. (You should not take licorice root if you have high blood pressure.)

Q: Which ones balance estrogen and which balance progesterone?

The ones that balance estrogen should be used if you are having scanty, irregular menses. These are alfalfa and red clover flowers and leaves, black cohosh root, hops, licorice root (don't use if you have high blood pressure), sage leaves, sweet briar hip or leaf buds, and pomegranate seeds.

The ones that balance progesterone should be used if you are bleeding copiously and frequently. These are chaste tree/Vitex berries, sarsaparilla root, wild yam root, and yarrow flowers and leaves.

Q: Can I make these herbs into a tea?

You can, but teas generally are too weak for medicinal purposes. A tea is usually a teaspoon of dried herb per cup of boiling water, steeped for five to fifteen minutes. The result is a light brew with not a great deal of plant nutrients in it.

Q: What is an infusion, and is it strong enough to work like medicine?

An infusion takes a greater quantity of herbal material than tea does (an ounce of roots or bark to a pint of water, an ounce of leaves or flowers to a quart of water) and steeps it for hours. The result is a dark liquid that can be kept for several days in the refrigerator.

An ounce of dried herb (roots, leaves, flowers, or seeds) is placed in a heatproof glass pint or quart jar and boiling water is poured in to cover the herb and fill the jar to the top. Then the jar is tightly closed and set aside to brew—the roots should be brewed for eight hours; the leaves for four hours; the flowers for two hours; and the seeds for half an hour. You can add honey or milk if the taste is too strong.

The brew is strong enough to work like medicine, taken internally. You can also use it externally for soaking or as a poultice.

Q: What is a tincture?

A tincture is made by steeping fresh plant material in alcohol. (If you are sensitive to alcohol, or prefer not to consume it, you can also buy tinctures that are steeped in vinegar, although the effect is somewhat weakened, and the product will not last as long.) Tinctures are readily available in health food stores, and they stay potent for years. You can make your own, although it's far easier to purchase common American brands. (European tinctures are not tested here and may not have the same quality and purity.)

Q: Do I use one herb at a time or several in combination?

Susun Weed, one of the most knowledgeable herbalists for women's health, recommends that you use one herb for two weeks each month for three or more months. If you select one and it's not doing anything for you, discontinue it and try another. You should take an infusion or tincture one to three times daily. Generally a cup contains 250 milliliters and is equivalent to around 20 drops of tincture.

Other Natural Methods for an Easier Menopause

If you are interested in a holistic program of health, you'll want to consider other methods of enhancing your endocrine system. Hatha yoga is one way to exercise the body's internal systems so that they function better; sex is another. You can also use visualization to picture yourself growing healthier and stronger day by day.

Q: What yoga exercises will stimulate my hormones?
The following exercises get a fresh input of blood flowing through the kidneys and adrenals. Yoga postures align the body in different ways so that various glands and internal organs get a good massage. Also, since you breathe deeply in each posture, you are able to send a fresh supply of oxygen directly to the tissues and cells you're targeting. (See Chapter 3 for a description of yoga and its importance for women in midlife.)

The upside-down dog: Get on your hands and knees and rest your palms on the floor in front of you. With feet flat on the floor, straighten your legs so that your body forms an inverted V. Breathe into the posture for a count of ten. When you are comfortable here, slide your forearms down so that they rest on the floor. Breathe for a count of ten.

The bridge: Lie on your back and bend your knees, putting your feet flat on the floor, about two feet apart. Push your hips into the air and rest the weight of your upper torso on your shoulders. Interlace your fingers on the floor below your back and breathe in the posture for a count of ten.

Head to knee posture: Sit with your legs apart. One leg is outstretched, and the other bent, the foot resting against the opposite inner thigh. Take a deep breath and bend over the outstretched leg, reaching for your ankle or foot. Hold the posture and don't bounce. Breathe deeply, feeling your hips and internal organs expand. Reverse legs and bend to the other side.

Q: How can sex stimulate my hormones?

When we are sexually aroused, our brain sends messages to the sexual organs to get us prepared for the moment of orgasm. Even when our bodies age, the Bartholin's glands above and on each side of the vaginal opening still produce natural secretions. And the more "practice" we have at lubricating, the better sex feels. Then, too, our tissues remain more elastic over time if we continue to engage in penetrative acts, from manual and oral activity to intercourse. Certain studies have shown that women with an active sex life have higher levels of estrogen than those who are celibate.

Q: How can I use visualization to increase my estrogen levels?

Sit quietly in a comfortable chair or cross-legged on the floor. Allow your mind to focus on your breath and enjoy the feeling of watching the inhalation and exhalation. As your breaths become deeper and fuller, imagine that they can propel you down inside your body to your pelvic cavity.

Now imagine your internal organs—see the barrel of your vagina, the relaxed bag of the uterus, the two gem-like ovaries held in the fingerlike projections at the top of the fallopian tubes.

Imagine that estrogen sits on these organs like dew on a field in the early morning. Your ovaries are plump with the hormone, as though it has just rained. You can see and feel the abundance. Know that any time you want more, you can direct your thoughts and feelings to this area and gather strength from it.

When you are ready, return to your regular breathing.

Become aware of your surroundings and allow your eyes to relax open.

Visualization works in a cumulative way—if you give yourself the time to do one of these daily or every other day, you'll find that you get the best effect from it.

Afterword

The next decades of your life could be exciting and challenging—or difficult and tedious. It all depends on you. If you are a person who always sees the glass as half full rather than half empty, you are going to be in good shape as you age. But even if it's hard for you right now to see yourself moving forward toward a great new future, you still have time to reassess your emotional needs and find a suitable path to get you where you need to go.

Midlife is a transition between the time when we concentrate on families, work, and achievements and the time when we move toward new personal goals and the great unknown of our old age. As such, it causes many problems and turns many lives upside down. It's harder to accept change as we grow older, yet many of us have to deal with forging new ways of coping, thinking, and being when we hit midlife.

This time of life is very similar to puberty, where you felt the first flush of what it meant to be a woman. You were excited and scared by it; drawn to it and repulsed by it. One day you were on top of the world—attractive and self-confident—the next day you wanted to crawl into a hole and disappear. A very similar set of feelings is triggered at midlife, when you are changing hormonally and may be going through major life changes at the same time.

But estrogen, important as it is to all of us, is only part of the answer. The rest of the questions, and the solutions you find, will lead you to discover what the world can give you and what you can give it, now that you've unlocked your true potential.

You've lived half your life. Make the rest even better.

Resource Guide for Women in Midlife

There is a wonderful network of help for midlife women, and if you know where to go and whom to ask, you'll be able to achieve the goals you set for yourself at this time of life. Because there are so many possibilities, you should read widely and diversely. Keep an open mind, whether you wish to consider hormones or alternative methods of dealing with your menopause.

National Organizations

The following groups are dedicated to disseminating helpful information to women all over the country on health care. They may be able to send you pamphlets and brochures relevant to your particular area of interest.

Planned Parenthood Federation of America
810 Seventh Avenue
New York, NY 10019
(212) 541-7800

Although Planned Parenthood's main thrust is counseling for women in their reproductive years, they are deeply committed to health care for midlife women as well. Their chapters all over the country offer counseling and gynecological care as well as carefully written and illustrated brochures on various medical conditions and surgical procedures.

American College of Obstetricians and Gynecologists
600 Maryland Avenue, S.W.
Washington, DC 20024
(202) 638-5577

For general information about menopause and a listing of physicians in your area.

National Self-Help Clearing House
33 W. 42 Street
New York, NY 10036
(212) 840-1259

Referrals to support groups; self-help newsletter.

The National Women's Health Network
1325 G Street, N.W.
Washington, DC 20005
(202) 347-1140

They will send a packet of resource materials for a $5 fee.

National Coalition on Older Women's Issues
2401 Virginia Avenue, N.W.
Washington, DC 20037
(202) 466-7834

Resource directory on midlife issues available for $4.

National Osteoporosis Foundation
2100 M Street, N.W.
Washington, DC 20037
1-800-223-9994

They publish a booklet called *Boning Up*, available by mail for $1, which discusses causes, treatment, and prevention of the disease.

North American Menopause Society
11100 Euclid Avenue
Cleveland, OH 44106
(216) 844-3334

Ongoing educational programs for women in midlife. The organization can also give you referrals to physicians in your area.

HERS (Hysterectomy Educational Resources and Services)
422 Bryn Mawr Avenue
Bala Cynwyd, PA 19004
(610) 667-7757

Educational brochures on hysterectomy and oophorectomy. This organization is devoted to the reduction in number of such surgeries.

Hotlines for Incontinence Problems

National Association for Continence (NAFC)
1-800-252-3337

Simon Foundation for Continence
1-800-237-4666

Vulvar Pain

Vulvar Pain Foundation
PO Drawer 177
Graham, NC 27252
(910) 226-0704

National Vulvodynia Association
PO Box 19288
Sarasota, FL 34276-2288
(941) 927-8503

Both organizations devoted to the treatment of vulvar pain offer educational brochures and can refer you to specialists in your area.

Libraries and Databases

The Internet can hook you up to medical libraries around the world, or if you're not computer savvy, you can order printouts from medical journals from the various resources listed below.

Grateful Med (a program available from the National Technical Information Service [NTIS] $29.95)
National Institutes of Health
National Library of Medicine
Bethesda, MD 20894
1-800-423-9255

Center for Medical Consumers/Health Care Library
237 Thompson Street
New York, NY 10012

An excellent resource for books and articles on conventional and alternative medicine. They also publish a monthly newsletter called *Healthfacts*.

World Research Foundation
15300 Ventura Boulevard, Suite 405
Sherman Oaks, CA 91403
(818) 907-5483

World Research will send you customized information packs on any health subject, complete with either conventional or alternative medical approaches, for $45 plus shipping.

Planetree Health Resource Center
2040 Webster Street
San Francisco, CA 94115
(415) 923-3681

You can get an in-depth information packet for $100, which offers a selection of the latest medical references, or you can simply order the $20 bibliography of sources and do the library or computer search yourself. They also have a directory of physicians and other health care practitioners, organizations, and support groups.

The Health Resource
Janice R. Guthrie
209 Katherine Drive
Conway, AR 72032
(501) 329-5272

This group will provide a complete set of reports on conventional or alternative treatment for medical problems for a fee of $195 plus shipping.

Women Helping Women

One of the best resources for information and support in this area are the many groups founded and run by women who've already been through menopause. Many offer emotional support; others offer counseling on issues ranging from medical problems to emotional health, finances, and social services. To find local support groups in your area, contact your YWCA, local hospitals, women's centers, and community colleges near you.

Resources for Midlife and Older Women
226 E. 70 Street, Suite 1C
New York, NY 10021
(212) 439-1913

Medical and psychological referrals.

O.W.L. (Older Women's League)
730 11 Street, N.W., Suite 300
Washington, DC 20001
(202) 783-6686
NYC Chapter: (212) 496-1409

This politically active group lobbies for equal opportunities for midlife and older women. There are local chapters all over the country. They will provide referrals to support groups and also publish a bimonthly newspaper, *The Owl Observer.*

Women's Helpline (NOW, NYC Service Fund)
15 W. 18 Street, 9th floor
New York, NY 10011
(212) 989-7230

Referrals to midlife women's groups and services.

Women's Action Alliance
370 Lexington Avenue, Room 603
New York, NY 10017
(212) 532-8330

Referrals for women in midlife.

Medical Help

If you feel that you are not getting the answers you need, or if you live near any of the following clinics, you will find excellent—although medicalized—care at any of the facilities listed below. Remember that the primary treatment of choice at these facilities will be hormone replacement therapy. The physicians will be board certified in gynecology or in endocrinology. There will be additional trained staff who are knowledgeable in areas as diverse as human sexuality, psychiatry, nutrition, and exercise.

Menopause Clinics

Cleveland Menopause Clinic
Mt. Sinai Medical Center
29001 Cedar Road, Suite 600
Lyndhurst, OH 44124
(216) 442-4747

The Climacteric Clinic, Women's Medical and
   Diagnostic Center
222 S.W. 36 Terrace, Suite C
University of Florida
Gainesville, FL 32607
(904) 372-5600

Menopause Clinic
Brigham and Women's Hospital
Fertility, Endocrine & Menopause Unit
75 Francis Street
Boston, MA 02115
(617) 732-4220

Menopause Center at UCLA
Center for Health Sciences, Department of Ob/Gyn
Room 22-177CHS
Los Angeles, CA 90024-1740
(213) 825-7755

UMDNJ–Robert Wood Johnson Medical School
Department of Obstetrics and Gynecology
1 Robert Wood Johnson Place–CN19
New Brunswick, NJ 08903–0019
(201) 937-7633

Menopause Care Center
George Washington University
2300 I Street, N.W.
Washington, DC 20037
(202) 994-5656

Menopause Clinic
Yale University School of Medicine
Physician's Building
Howard Avenue
New Haven, CT 06520
(203) 785-4708

Menopausal Section
Baylor Ob/Gyn
6550 Fannin Street
Houston, TX 77030
(713) 798-7500

Menopause Clinic
University of San Diego Medical Center
225 Dickenson Street
San Diego, CA 92103
Clinic phone: (619) 543-3210
Hot flash phone: (619) 453-3210 (A nurse from the
   clinic will give you immediate information.)

Northwest Memorial Faculty Foundation
Department of Reproductive Endocrinology
680 N. Lakeshore Drive, Suite 810
Chicago, IL 60611
(312) 908-7269

Menopause Clinic
University of Illinois Hospital and Clinics
840 S. Wood, Room 13 Yellow
Chicago, IL 60612
(312) 996-6870

Non–Drug-Related Treatment

If you are interested in any of the holistic methods of
dealing with menopause, see Chapter 9 for instructions on
finding a qualified practitioner. You may also wish to write
to the various national organizations for referrals.

Nutrition

American Dietetic Association
216 W. Jackson Boulevard, Suite 800
Chicago, IL 60606
(312) 899-0040

Center for Science in the Public Interest
1501 16 Street, N.W.
Washington, DC 20036
(202) 332-9110

Herbalism

You may write to the companies below for a catalogue
and price list:

Avena Botanicals
PO Box 365
West Rockport, ME 04865

Blessed Herbs
Route 5, Box 1042
Ava, MO 65608

Herb Pharm
Box 116
Williams, OR 97544

Wish Garden Herbs
PO Box 1304
Boulder, CO 80306

Homeopathy

International Foundation for Homeopathy
2366 East Lake E., 301
Seattle, WA 98102
(206) 324-8230

National Center for Homeopathy
1500 Massachusetts Avenue, N.W.
Washington, DC 20005
(202) 223-6182

Hypnosis

American Association of Professional Hypnotherapists
PO Box 731
McLean, VA 22101
(703) 448-9623

American Society of Clinical Hypnosis
2250 E. Devon Avenue, Suite 336
Des Plaines, IL 60018
(312) 297-3317

Chiropractic

American Chiropractic Association
1091 Wilson Boulevard
Arlington, VA 22201
(703) 276-8800

Biofeedback

Association for Applied Psychophysiology and
   Biofeedback
10200 W. 44 Avenue
Wheat Ridge, CO 80033
(303) 422-8434

The association can provide you with lists of hospitals where you can get biofeedback training, private licensed practitioners, and information about the technique and its use.

Self-Care Catalogue (biofeedback equipment for
   urinary incontinence)
5850 Shellmound Avenue
Emeryville, CA 94662-0813

Vaginal Weights

Femina Vaginal Weights (for Kegel practice)
Dacomed Corporation
1701 E. 79 Street
Minneapolis, MN 55425

Light Therapy

Society for Light Treatment and Biological Rhythm
722 W. 168 Street
Box 50
New York, NY 10032

Alternative Care

Dr. Fredi Kronenberg
The Richard and Hinda Rosenthal Center for
    Alternative/Complementary Medicine
Columbia University College of Physicians and
    Surgeons
630 W. 168 Street
New York, NY 10032
(212) 305-4755

Wise Woman Center
PO Box 64
Woodstock, NY 12498

Prescriptions for "Natural" Hormones

Here is a list of pharmacies that supply natural estrogen
and progesterone products.

Bajamar Women's Healthcare Pharmacy
9609 Dielman Rock Island
St. Louis, MO 63132
1-800-255-8025

Belmar Pharmacy
12860 W. Cedar Drive, #210
Lakewood, CO 80228
(303) 763-5533

Bezwecken Transdermal Systems
12525 S.W. 3 Street
Beaverton, OR 97005
1-800-243-2256

College Pharmacy
833 N. Tejom
Colorado Springs, CO 80903
1-800-888-9358

Delk Pharmacy
1602 Hatcher Lane
Columbia, TN 38401
(615) 388-3952

Lloyd Center Pharmacy
1302 Lloyd Center
Portland, OR 97232
1-800-358-8974

Madison Pharmacy Associates
429 Gammon Place
Madison, WI 53719
1-800-558-7046

Medical Center Pharmacy
10721 Main Street
Fairfax, VA 22030
1-800-723-7455

Transitions to Health
621 S.W. Alder, #900
Portland, OR 97205-3267
1-800-888-6814

Wellness Pharmacy
2800 S. 18 Street
Birmingham, AL 35209
1-800-227-2627

Women's International Pharmacy
5709 Monona Drive
Madison, WI 53716-3152
1-800-279-5708

Recommended Reading

Women and Midlife

Barbach, Lonnie. *The Pause*. New York: Dutton, 1993.

Boston Women's Health Book Collective. *The New Our Bodies, Ourselves*. New York: Simon & Schuster, 1992.

Brown, Lyn Mikel, and Carol Gilligan. *Meeting at the Crossroads: Turning Points in Girls' and Women's Lives*. New York: Ballantine Books, 1992.

Cobb, Janine O'Leary. *Answers and Advice for Women in the Prime of Life*. New York: Plume, 1993.

Cutler, Winnifred B. *Hysterectomy, Before and After*. New York: Harper & Row, 1988.

———. *Love Cycles: The Science of Intimacy*. New York: Villard Books, 1991.

Doress, Paula B., and Diana L. Siegal, eds. *Ourselves Growing Older*. Rev. ed. Midlife and Older Women's Book Project. New York: Simon & Schuster, 1992.

Dranov, Paula. *Estrogen: Is It Right for You?* New York: Fireside Press, 1993.

Greenwood, Sadja. *Menopause Naturally*. Updated. San Francisco: Volcano Press, 1992.

Greer, Germaine. *The Change: Women, Aging, and the Menopause*. New York: Knopf, 1991.

Hall, Judy, and Dr. Robert Jacobs. *The Wise Woman*. Rockport, MA: Element, Inc., 1992.

Jacobowitz, Ruth. *The 150 Most Asked Questions About Menopause*. New York: Hearst Books, 1993.

Lark, Susan. *The Menopause Self-Help Book*. Berkeley, CA: Celestial Arts Press, 1990.

McCain, Marian Van Eyk. *Transformation Through Menopause*. New York: Bergin & Garvey, 1991.

Nachtigall, Lila, M.D., and Joan Rattner Heilman. *Estrogen: The Facts Can Change Your Life*. New York: HarperCollins, 1995.

National Women's Health Network Staff. *Taking Hormones and Women's Health: Choices, Risks, Benefits*. Rev. ed. Washington, D.C., 1995.

Nissim, Rina. *Natural Healing in Gynecology*. New York: Pandora Press, 1984.

Perry, Susan, and Katherine O'Hanlan. *Natural Menopause*. Reading, MA.: Addison Wesley, 1992.

Porcino, Jane. *Growing Older, Getting Better*. New York: Crossroad Publishing Co., 1991.

Reitz, Rosetta. *Menopause: A Positive Approach*. New York: Penguin Books, 1981.

Sachs, Judith. *What Women Should Know About Menopause*. New York: Dell, 1991.

————. *The Healing Power of Sex*. Englewood Cliffs, NJ: Prentice Hall, 1994.

Sachs, Judith, and Elizabeth Ross, M.D. *Healing the Female Heart*. New York: Pocket Books, 1996.

Sarrel, Phillip, M.D. *Sexual Turning Points.* New York: Macmillan, 1984.

Sheehy, Gail. *The Silent Passage.* New York: Random House, 1991.

Starr, Bernard D., Ph.D., and Marcella Bakur Weiner, Ed.D. *On Sex and Sexuality in the Mature Years.* New York: Stein & Day, 1981.

Tavris, Carol. *Th. Mismeasure of Woman.* New York: Simon & Schuster, 1992.

Taylor, Dena, and Amber Sumrall, eds. *Women of the 14th Moon: Writing on Menopause.* Freedom, CA.: The Crossing Press, 1991.

Utian, Wulf H., and Ruth S. Jacobowitz. *Managing Your Menopause.* Englewood Cliffs, NJ: Prentice Hall, 1990.

Weed, Susun S. *The Menopausal Years.* Woodstock, N.Y.: Ash Tree Publishing, 1992.

Aging

Adler, Lynn. *Centenarians: People over 100—A Triumph of Will and Spirit.* Sante Fe, NM: Health Press, 1993.

Baltes, Paul B., and Margaret M. Baltes. *Successful Aging: Perspectives from the Behavioral Sciences.* New York: Cambridge University Press, 1993.

Banner, Lois W. *In Full Flower: Aging Women, Power and Sexuality.* New York: Random House, 1993.

Blair, Cornelia, Mark A. Siegel, and Nancy R. Jacobs. *Growing Old in America.* Rev. ed. Wylie, TX: Information Plus, 1994.

Booth, Wayne C., ed. *The Art of Growing Older: Writers on Living and Aging.* New York: Poseidon Press, 1992.

Bortz, Walter M., II, M.D. *We Live Too Short and Die Too Long.* New York: Bantam Books, 1991.

Burton, Linda, ed. *Families and Aging.* Amityville, NY: Baywood Publishing Co., 1993.

Cole, Thomas R. *The Journey of Life: A Cultural History of Aging in America.* New York: Cambridge University Press, 1992.

Coni, Nicholas, William Davison, and Stephen Webster. *Aging: The Facts.* 2d ed. New York: Oxford University Press, 1992.

Dass, Ram. *Conscious Aging: On the Nature of Change and Facing Death.* 1993. (Two cassettes.)

Dow, Alastair. *Deprenyl: The Anti-Aging Drug.* Tampa, FL: Hallberg Publishing Corp., 1993.

Edelman, Deborah S. *Sex in the Golden Years: What's Ahead May Be Worth Aging For.* New York: Donald I. Fine, Inc., 1992.

Evans, Williams, and Irwin Rosenberg, M.D. *Biomarkers: The 10 Determinants of Aging.* New York: Simon & Schuster, 1991.

Friedan, Betty. *The Fountain of Age.* New York: Simon & Schuster, 1993.

Fries, James, and Lawrence Crapo. *Vitality and Aging.* San Francisco: Freeman, 1981.

Gardner, John. *Self-Renewal.* New York: Norton, 1981.

Glasse, Lou, and Jon Hendricks, eds. *Gender and Aging: Generations and Aging.* Amityville, NY: Baywood Publishing Co., 1992.

Lieberman, Florence, and Morris F. Collen. *Aging in Good Health: A Quality Lifestyle for the Later Years.* New York: Plenum Publishing, 1993.

Mollen, Art, and Judith Sachs. *Dr. Mollen's Anti-Aging Diet.* New York: NAL/Dutton, 1992.

Stokes, Lydia. *The Longevity Factor.* New York: HarperCollins, 1993.

Thomas, Lewis. *The Medusa and the Snail: More Notes of a Biology Watcher.* New York: Viking Press, 1977.

Newsletters

A Friend Indeed
Box 1710
Champlain, NY 12919-1710
(514) 843-5730
Subscription is $30 a year for 10 issues.

Midlife Woman
5129 Logan Avenue South
Minneapolis, MN 55419-1019
(612) 925-0020
Subscription is $25 a year for 6 issues.

Wellness Newsletter (Johns Hopkins Medical School)
PO Box 420235
Palm Coast, FL 32142-0235
1-800-829-9170
Subscription is $24 a year for 12 issues.

Harvard Women's Health Watch
164 Longwood Avenue
Boston, MA 02115
1-800-829-5921
Subscription is $32 a year for 12 issues.

Index